THE *good* **SEX** *guide* ABROAD

The author would like to thank Rita Ward and Colette Batterby at the International Planned Parenthood Federation Library, and Margaret McGovern and Toni Belfield from the Family Planning Association for their invaluable help and support in preparing this book.

THIS IS A CARLTON BOOK

THIS EDITION PUBLISHED IN 1995 BY BCA BY ARRANGEMENT WITH CARLTON BOOKS LIMITED

Copyright © Carlton Books Limited 1995

All rights reserved.

This book is sold subject to the condition that it shall not, by way of trade or otherwise, be lent, resold, hired out or otherwise circulated without the publisher's prior written consent in any form of cover or binding other than that in which it is published and without a similar condition including this condition being imposed upon the subsequent purchaser.

CN 9879

Executive Editor: Lorraine Dickey
Art Direction: Russell Porter
Design: Fiona Knowles
Project Editor: Ann Kay
Photography: Paul Matlock
Illustrations: Jo Hall, Jackie Harland,
   Debbie Hinks, Dannie Alex Weir
Picture Research: Charlotte Bush
Production: Garry Lewis

Printed in Italy

THE good SEX guide ABROAD

Techniques from around the world
to add sparkle to your sex life

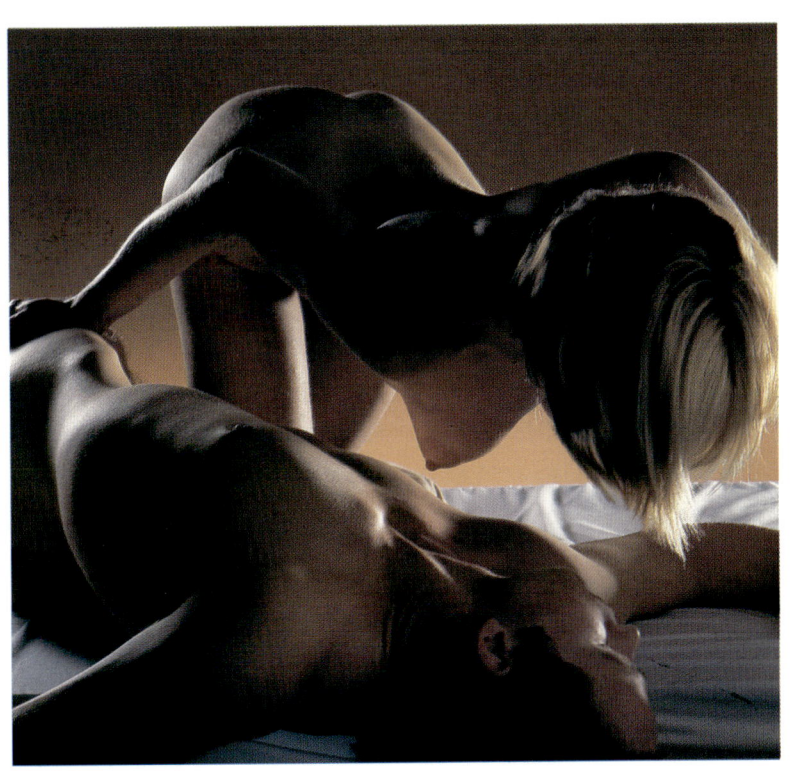

SUZIE HAYMAN

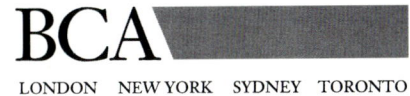

LONDON NEW YORK SYDNEY TORONTO

Contents

Foreword   6

1 What's Sexy   8

2 Love, Courtship & Marriage   26

3 Sex Techniques & Practices   42

4 Sexual Positions   66

5 Sex Aids   88

6 Vive les differences   112

Index   126

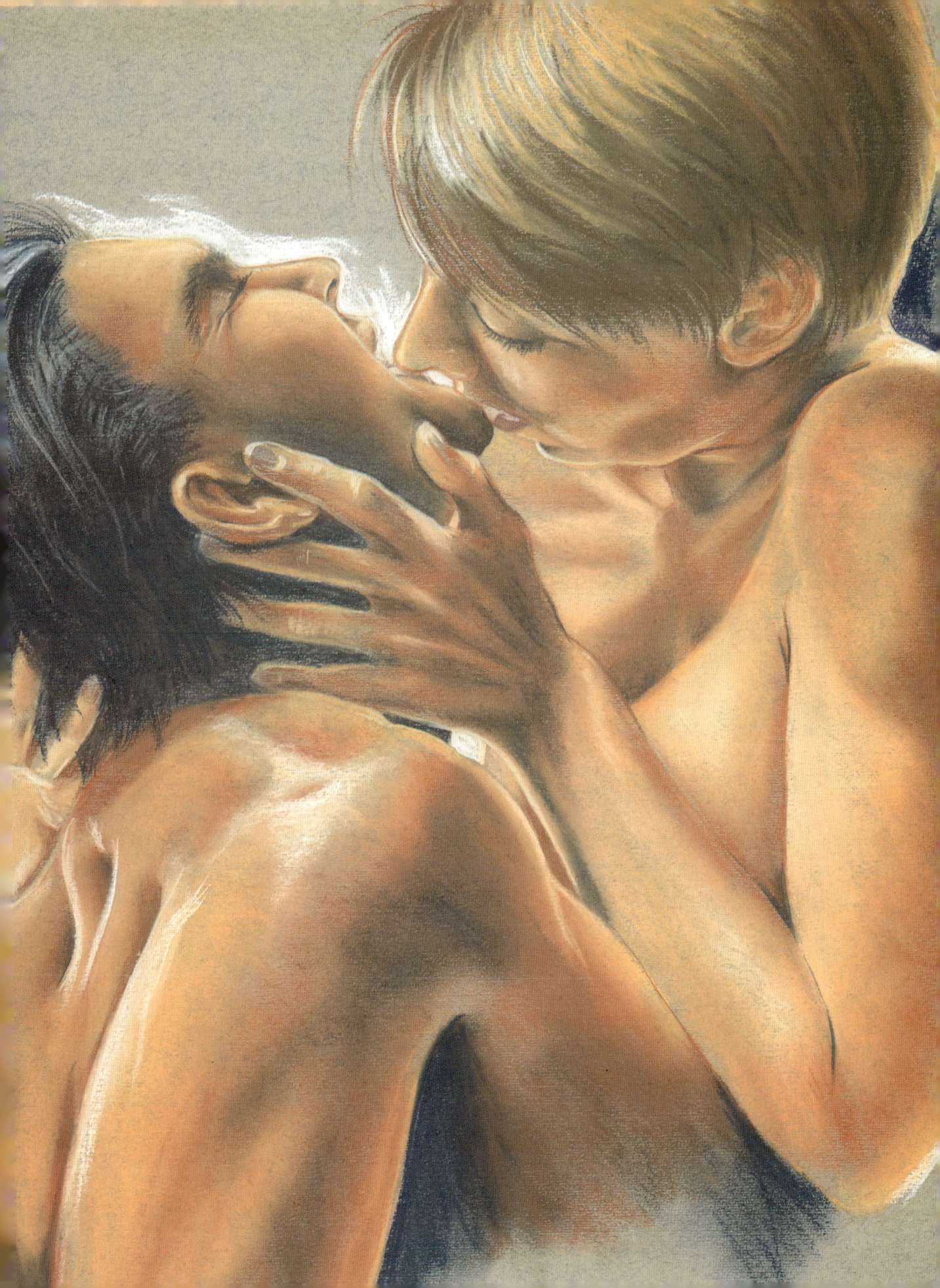

Foreword

They said I had the best job in television, presenting *The Good Sex Guide*, and then they sent me around the world to have a look at how everyone else does it. I thought I'd died and gone to heaven.

Did you know that every day around the world over 50 million people are at it! That's a whole lot of loving and there's plenty of variation right round the globe. There's over 800 different cultural groups in the world and all of them with different tips to pass on. Some people believe you can even tell what a person will be like in bed by looking at their face and body! Look out for men with big noses and wide nostrils, girls – but the news there is not all good!

The customs and beliefs that govern our sexual behaviour means that in some countries sex is spiritual and sacred, whilst in others sex takes place with your mother-in-law in the room! I don't think that would go down a bundle in Speke.

Another thing that fascinated me was discovering that sexual practices which are taboo in some societies are completely acceptable in others. I started to wish I'd been born in a warmer climate. Did you know a proper French kiss can burn off up to 12 calories? And as you would expect, sexual experimentation in the Western world has led to the adoption of many ideas imported from the East – can't say they've taken many of ours though!

What does seem universal is that most people want passionate and meaningful sex. Particularly if it involves hours of foreplay as well as multiple orgasms and a cosmic oneness with your partner! It's also clear that obsessions are the same the world over. Obsession with the performance and size of penis that is!

I hope this book helps you develop a deeper understanding of the wonderful world of sex. It's essential if you want to know why our definition of what's sexy is seen as a total turn-off elsewhere round the globe.

Ta Ra

Margi

What's Sexy?

1

Sex makes the world go round and although we speak different languages, have different customs and even different appearances, one thing is constant in every race. That's the fact that we all do it, we all like doing it and much of our time is spent thinking how, when and with whom we are going to do it next!

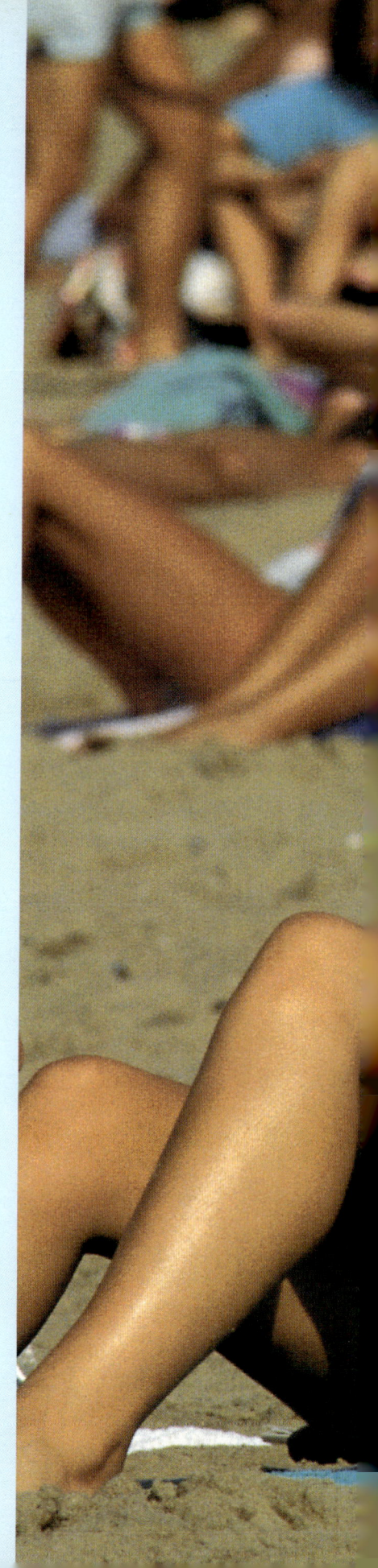

An all-over tan, long legs, blond hair and well-sized, firm breasts with erect nipples are what makes a woman attractive in Western eyes

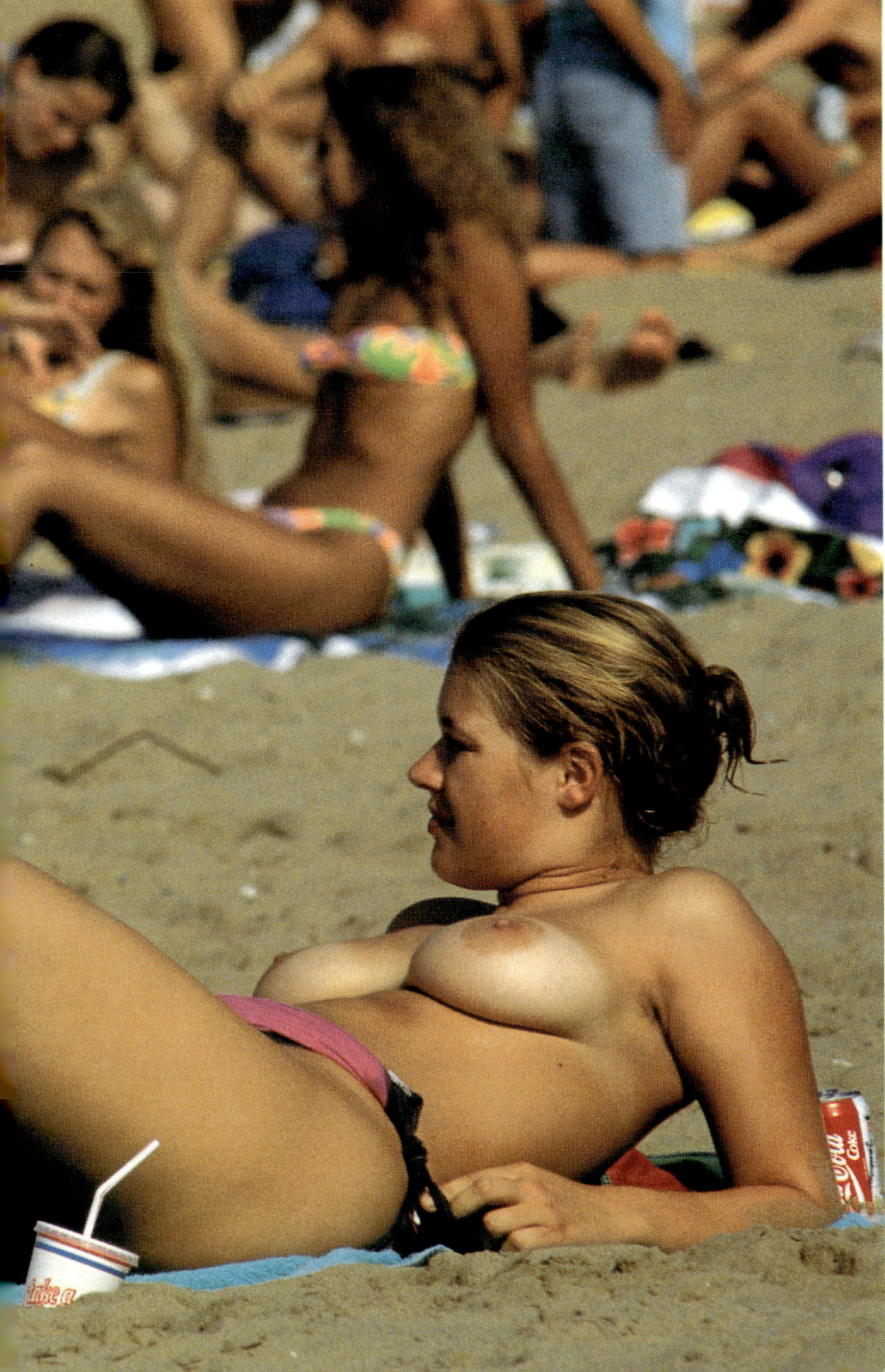

You probably have a pretty firm idea of what makes a man or a woman sexually desirable. In Western society, sex appeal tends to come from tanned skin, firm breasts or pecs, tight buttocks, long legs, and white, even teeth. Men and women show off what they've got in tight jeans and revealing tops, and with careful use of cosmetic products. Dieting and fitness can be major preoccupations. But if you think that the standards of sexual attraction are universal, you would be wrong. Every society has a different idea of what is sexually desirable. An ample backside, breasts that hang low and blackened teeth may be the very last word in drop-dead attractiveness to different groups of people across the globe.

All societies, however, share an interest in how bodies are displayed and the sexual signals that our bodies send out to other people. The display is pretty obvious in the West, where clothes, art and the mass media seem totally engaged in sending sexual messages. Messages may be more subtle in Eastern societies, but they're still there. Even societies with apparently negative attitudes towards sexuality have a preoccupation with sex in reality. After all, spending a lot of time insisting that you shouldn't be sending out sexual messages means you are thinking about it just as much as if you were!

TELLING LOOKS

But before we even look at the different styles in various societies, are there any sexual characteristics that are recognizable throughout the whole human race? Can you tell what a person may be like in bed simply by looking at their face or body?

There is a common belief in the West that the size of a man's penis is indicated by the size of his nose. If you ask women – and men – to pick from a group of pictures the men they think are sexy, those with strong, aquiline noses tend to be chosen. Similarly, a woman's vagina is supposed to match her mouth, and women with wide, generous mouths are often selected.

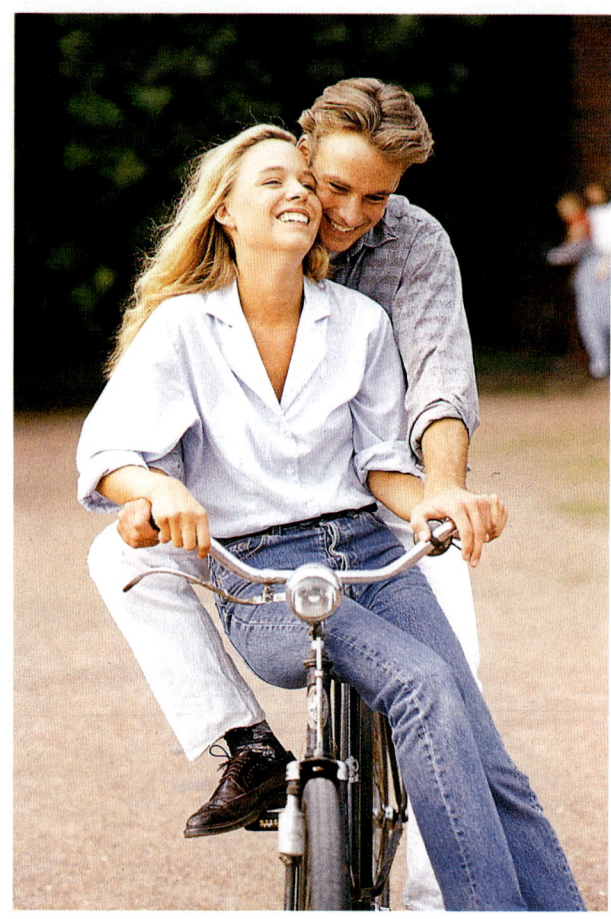

THIS IS THE PERFECT COUPLE AS FAR AS MOST WESTERNERS ARE CONCERNED – TALL, SLENDER AND FAIR, WITH GLEAMING WHITE SMILES AND A GENERAL AIR OF HEALTH AND FITNESS

The Chinese agree with this, and also believe that you can interpret a person's character, and particularly their sexual characteristics, from their looks. A man with a big nose and wide nostrils is expected to have a strong penis but to lack stamina when making love. Someone with a wide philtrum (the groove that goes from the base of the nose to the upper lip) will have a lusty sexual appetite. A woman with a small mouth and a thin upper lip will orgasm quickly. Rounded chins are the sign of passion and sexual enthusiasm, while long, thick upper lips in either sex show that the person is slow to arouse, slow to come and slow to give satisfaction to their partner.

However, none of the scientific studies published substantiate these myths, nor do they confirm the idea that penis size differs between races. When Alfred Kinsey, the American sex researcher, conducted the largest study of penile size ever done, he found an enormous range, going from 3.8 cm to 16.5 cm (when flaccid), among both white and non-white men.

COMPATIBLE PARTS

Various societies classify men and women according to their body types or their sexual organs. Hindu genital classification, as described in the ancient text on the arts of love, the *Kama Sutra*, says that there are three types of penis, and three types of vagina. Hindus believe there are three couplings that will be equal, where the couple will have no sexual problems, and six where inequality could give you something to worry about.

According to the *Kama Sutra*, men are divided into Hares, Bulls and Horses. Hares have penes up to 6 finger-widths in length when erect. Bulls go up to 9 finger-widths and Horses up to 12. Among women, there are Deer, Mares and Elephants. Deer women have vaginas that are 6 finger-widths deep, Mares are 9 and Elephants are up to 12. According to this belief, if a Hare man makes love to an Elephant woman, she won't feel a thing. While if a Horse tries to cosy up to a Deer, she's going to feel it's all too much for her. Some of the sexual positions described in the *Kama Sutra* are specifically designed to overcome these problems. (We'll talk more about that in Chapter 4.)

DIFFERENT STROKES
FOR DIFFERENT FOLKS

Indian love manuals also describe women as falling into four distinct types. There are Lotus women, who like to make love in the daytime, and are full-breasted, soft and very beautiful. The Artistic women are similar in appearance, but like to make love at night and are experts in the sensual arts, while Conch women are earthier than the first two types, have smaller breasts and larger bodies, and are likely to have sudden bouts of passion. Finally, there are the Elephant women, who are slow, short and plump and like to take their love for hours at a time.

An American psychologist called William Sheldon, working in the 1940s, said that, while people did not fit into rigid categories of body type, there were three basic structural tendencies, which he called Endomorph, Mesomorph and Ectomorph. He also associated these with certain personality traits and sexual behaviours, as you can see in the box "Sheldon's body-typing", on page 12. However, Sheldon suggested that these classifications were variable, and that most people were on the borderline, taking characteristics from two types. So there's no reason to assume that the hunk with dynamite pecs or the girl with all those curves are necessarily boring in bed!

SOME SEX POSITIONS MAY NEED FLEXIBILITY AND PLENTY OF PRACTICE TO GET THEM RIGHT, BUT CHANCES ARE THEY COULD BE BOTH FUN AND HIGHLY SATISFYING

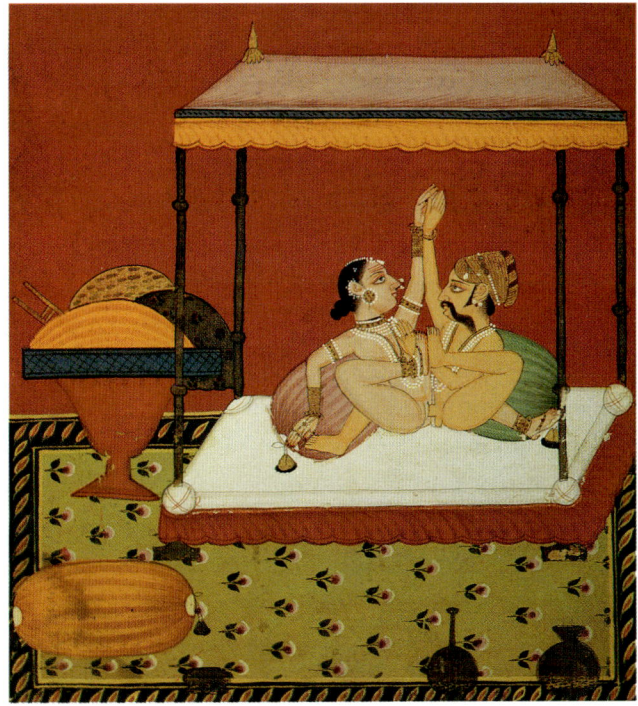

Sheldon's body-typing

The ENDOMORPH has a round, soft and heavy body and tends to be sociable, easy-going and pleasure-loving. Endomorphs have a great need for companionship but a lesser appetite for sex. MESOMORPHS are muscular, athletic, physically active and ready for action. They tend to be rather unimaginative and matter-of-fact about sex. The ECTOMORPH is tall and thin and has a restrained, inward-looking and sensitive personality. Every so often ectomorphs are overwhelmed with sexual desire and experience the most intense ecstasy when it is satisfied.

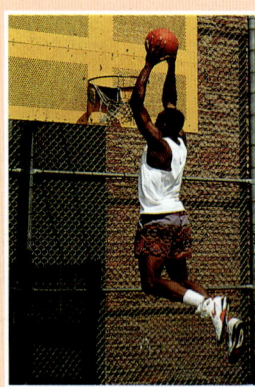
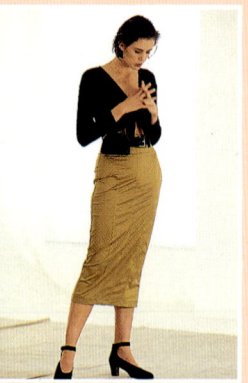
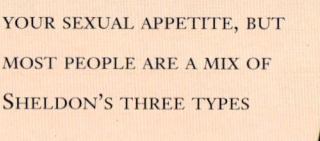

YOUR BODY SHAPE MAY SUGGEST YOUR SEXUAL APPETITE, BUT MOST PEOPLE ARE A MIX OF SHELDON'S THREE TYPES

THE BODY BEAUTIFUL

It's a sad fact that most people in the West, men and women, dislike at least some part of their body. Many sexual and relationship problems stem from the sort of low self-esteem that often shows itself as dissatisfaction with our bodies. This obsession with body image in the West is easy to understand when you consider the media messages that are pumped out every day. Commercial image-makers use the body beautiful to sell everything from cars to lavatory cleaners, and at the same time are also selling us a concept of the ideal body. In the white, Western world this ideal usually has to be tall, slim and tanned. If it's a woman, it has to have long hair on the head but be depilated on legs, arms and armpits. She will be blessed with medium-sized, apple-shaped breasts with erect nipples. Her media man-mate will have a sprinkling of masculine hair on his body and a nicely sized, evenly shaped lunch-box in his trousers.

In the USA, a recent survey showed that over 90% of white women expressed dissatisfaction with their bodies. A massive 83% thought that dieting was necessary, even though nearly two thirds of those interviewed were in a weight range considered to be medically acceptable. Perhaps the most disturbing finding was that the women interviewed were almost united in what they saw to be the desirable ideal body – a five foot seven inch woman weighing just over 100 pounds. This is a perfect, scaled-up description of the sort of plastic doll whose image has been haunting the ideas of young girls for the last 35 years. In real life, anyone with a body like this wouldn't be able to have periods, or probably to have a sex-life with anything other than another plastic doll!

However, this ideal is actually a fairly rare preferred body type among societies elsewhere. If you consider the huge range of female types that are delighted in around the world every day, you can see that whatever figure you have, someone, somewhere, loves it. Take, for instance, the first real pin-up. Born about 25,000 years ago, during the last ice age, the "Venus of Willendorf" and her sisters would have been down at their local shopping mall looking for size 30 dresses and 44GG bras. Big was definitely beautiful and little has changed in many societies. Farming and foraging peoples see the good sense of carrying your foodstore around with you. This love of the big among communities with unreliable food supplies still exists today in certain tribal groups.

THIN HAS NOT ALWAYS BEEN THOUGHT BEAUTIFUL. MANY ANCIENT CARVINGS AND STATUES TELL A DIFFERENT STORY

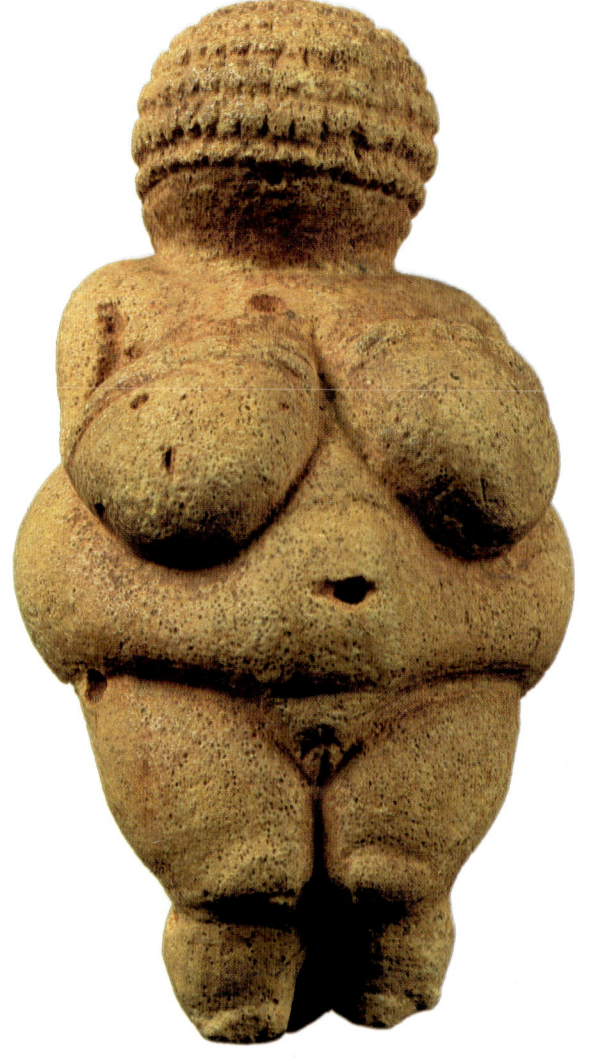

> ## What are your good bits?
>
> *Strip naked and stand in front of a mirror. Now, have a long, hard look at your body – but be honest rather than critical. Pretend it isn't your body, but that of a friend, and tell your friend which bits he or she has that are attractive. Forget the media hype about skinny supermodels or pumped-up weightlifters. What are your good bits? You will find that you have plenty, if you only bother to look properly.*

The Marquesans, in the central Pacific, think the most flattering thing you can say about a girl is to call her *tau, tau*, which means "fat". The liking of a bit of flesh has always been fashionable, if for no other reason than it has been quite correctly seen as an indication of potential fertility. Some substance on a body's bones is also healthier and provides better resistance to illness than skinniness. Artists through the ages, who have always had a free choice of the type of nude women they portrayed, have almost exclusively plumped for a bit of padding.

Outside the West, only the Yakut of north-eastern Siberia prefer their women slim. In virtually every other society, weight and sexual attractiveness go together. In some, particularly in Africa, plumpness is so important as a desirable quality for a bride, that women must be fattened up before being married. The ceremony can only go ahead if the bride is sufficiently large!

There are countless examples of lusty praise being heaped on ample women. Consider this extract from the unexpurgated *Arabian Nights*: "...her backside, dimpled with valleys, was so remarkable a benediction that she could not move easily without it trembling like curdled milk in a Badawi's porringer or quince jelly heaped on a plate perfumed with benzoin." A big bum, indeed!

Part of the obsession with fat in the West may have a lot to do with the way young people learn about sex and growing up. In societies where sex talk is fairly open, children know what to expect when their bodies alter at puberty. As a layer of subcutaneous padding fills out their outlines and genitals alter in size, shape and texture, Western women may be alarmed and confused. The result can be a horror at what is seen as "fat", and an obsession with attempts to get back to the child-like outline they once had.

A famous American woman once said "You can never be too rich or too thin," but consider the real tastes of the humble Western male. An American survey showed that most men would prefer their partners to be 10% overweight than 10% underweight. It seems likely that the majority of men would side with the 19th-century French writer Théophile Gautier when he says, when describing his ideal kind of woman, "I should scarcely like to meet a corner when I expected a circumference."

Ask your partner

You may have firm views about your body, but have you ever asked your partner what they think, and really listened to the answer? Men are often convinced that their partners want muscles, hairy chests and a bulging packet. Women are mostly sure their lovers are only turned on by big breasts and tiny waists. But what if he really prefers "something to get hold of" and dreams of a backside he needs a mountaineering axe to climb over? And what if she goes for the shy, slim, academic look rather than the hunk? Ask your partner what they really like, and what bits of you actually fulfil their fantasies. You may be very pleasantly surprised!

Even in North America, while 90% of white women were dissatisfied and diet-crazy, 70% of black women were satisfied with their shape and saw little reason to change. The essential difference in the two attitudes may rest in the fact that there is a relative absence of black women in the media. This means there are no unrealistic, "thin" ideals to live up to, leaving natural and cultural patterns as the ones to aspire to.

THE REAR VIEW

Whether you call them a bum, a fanny or a Khyber Pass, the buttocks have always been a prime focus for eyes, hands and the longing wolf whistle. It is hardly surprising, therefore, to find out that the muscles that make up these wondrous orbs are the largest in the human body. Because your backside contains so much muscle, it means that this is one part of your sexual equipment that you *can* improve dramatically by your own efforts. So give it the regular exercise it deserves.

Rounded buttocks have always been a female "gender signal" – a physical clue that enables us to identify an individual as male or female. Female baboons go in for obvious signals, and during mating periods their bottoms swell up to several times their normal size and take on rainbow colours. Human females make the same signals artificially, as they dance the night away dressed in skin-tight, multi-coloured lycra. Most women start building their ideal man from a firm little bottom, and only then add the other less tactile qualities like nice eyes and a sense of humour. Men share this fascination with the well-shaped derrière, and its presence is probably the only reason they are ever happy to have a lover walk away from them.

Which bits of their bodies do most Westerners feel have let them down? Weak chins, big noses and protruding teeth may feature, but it is breasts in women and the size, shape and appearance of

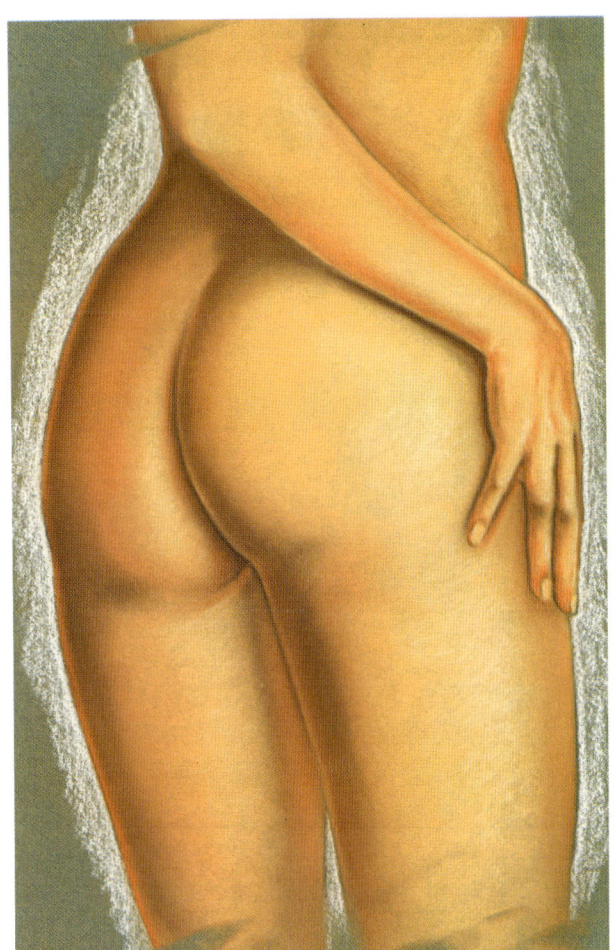

A WELL-SHAPED DERRIERE, WHETHER IT BE AN AMPLE FEMALE BEHIND OR A PERT AND TIGHT MALE BUTT, SENDS OUT EXTREMELY POWERFUL SIGNALS TO POTENTIAL SEXUAL PARTNERS

the genitals in both sexes that are the greatest causes of heartache.

Women are frequently convinced that their breasts are the wrong size and shape, particularly too small, slack or soft. Nipples are often felt to be inadequate if they are soft more often than erect or are surrounded by hair. Female woe will also be caused by stretchmarks or any visible veins. Are these universal worries?

The Zulu, from South Africa, have a custom in which unmarried women dance wearing nothing but beads, to show that their breasts are still firm and round. Flattened breasts are believed to be a sign of sexual immorality. Breasts soften as you get older and after breastfeeding, so it would be true that this could be a sign of having had children – in many cultures an unacceptable state for an unmarried girl! But other cultures, such as the Zande from the Sudan region, idealize long, hanging breasts. They prefer older women, seeing experience and maturity as desirable qualities.

THE FEMALE BREAST

Breasts may be Nature's way of providing a ready-mixed meal at exactly the right temperature but, as far as many people the world over are concerned, their main function is sexual and ornamental.

The female breast is made up of a network of milk-producing ducts surrounded by supportive tissue and pads of fat. The amount of fat tends to be related to a woman's general build. A slim woman is likely to have small, firm breasts. One with a generous build will have larger, softer breasts. Whatever their build, it's common for women to have one breast larger than the other and for their shape and texture to be different. Most breasts are covered, as is the rest of the body, with fine, downy hair. This can often be longer and darker nearer the nipple, forming a ring of long hairs.

The breasts contain no muscle at all, which is why no amount of exercise or therapy will increase their size. There is, however, a sheet of muscle – the pectoral muscle – which lies between the breast and the chest wall. This can indeed be firmed and enlarged by exercise, providing a firmer platform from which the breasts can hang, but having no effect on breast size itself. Pregnancy and breastfeeding, of course, will often increase their size as milk-producing tissue and fat stores increase. Size increase can also come with use of the oral contraceptive pill, because it mimics the hormone levels present in a pregnant woman and stimulates the milk ducts.

When a breastfeeding mum has weaned her child, the breasts return to their former size, the

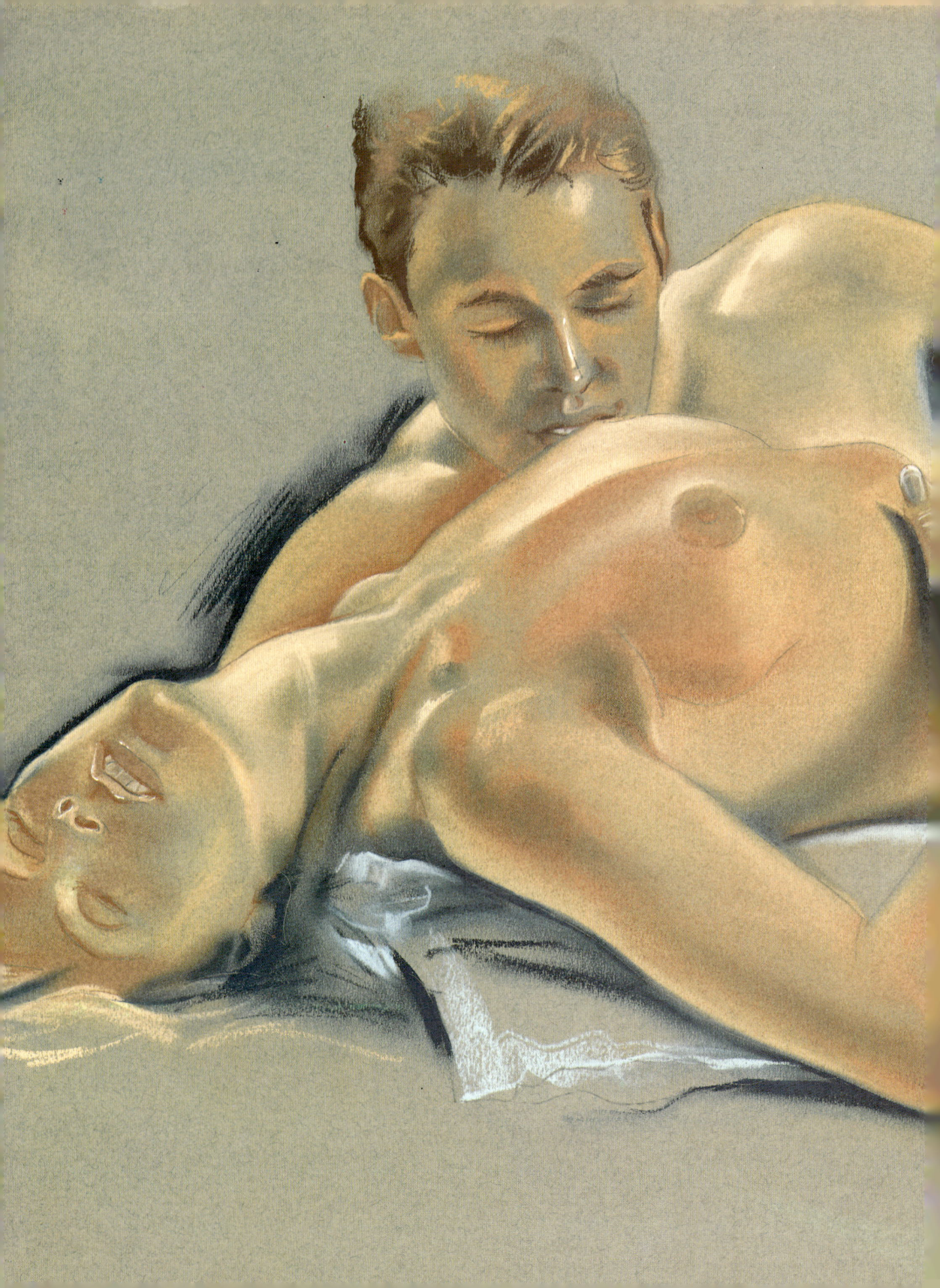

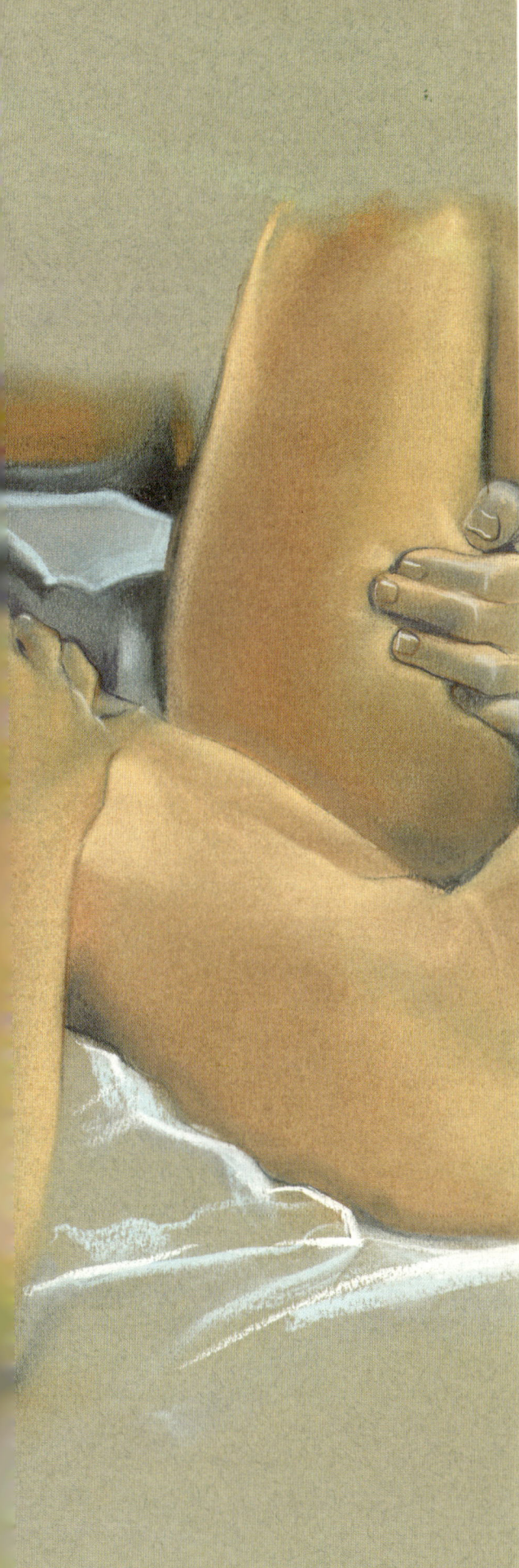

WOMEN ARE OFTEN WORRIED ABOUT WHAT MEN WILL THINK OF THEIR BREASTS. THE TRUTH IS, FEW MEN CAN RESIST THEM, WHATEVER THEIR SIZE AND SHAPE

extra fat having been converted to energy. Faint, silvery lines called stria will mark the increase and decrease in size. These are caused by bundles of fibres under the skin having been stretched and broken, so creams, oils or lotions massaged into the surface will have absolutely no effect on their appearance.

As women age, the fibrous breast tissues slacken. After menopause, the milk ducts shrink, and the whole breast can become smaller and softer. In some cases, fat replaces these tissues, so overall size is not lost but firmness will almost certainly lessen.

A more short-lived change in a woman's breasts is produced by sexual stimulation, when the whole chest area can become mottled and the veins become dramatically visible. Just before orgasm, the breast may swell by as much as a quarter.

Breasts get a 10 out of 10 rating for erotic potential in most men's and women's priorities. Very few men of any culture are indifferent to them, although not all demand that they be large and firm. The sensation of rubbing your hand over a silky globe that yields to the touch, and the satisfaction and reassurance that comes when this area visibly reacts in excitement, make a woman's breasts one of her lover's first targets. Similarly, few women find the sensation of having their breasts caressed unpleasant, to say the least.

NIPPLES

Nipples are made of erectile tissue that fills with blood and becomes firm and stands out under stimulus. The stimulus can be sexual excitement, fear, physical exertion, cold or just the sensation of being rubbed, for instance by loose clothing. Some women have nipples that turn inwards and will only erect when actually manipulated out by your own or your lover's fingertips.

When a woman is sexually stimulated, nipples erect and the surrounding area flushes a darker colour. During lovemaking, nipples do not simply erect and remain rock-hard. They fluctuate, softening and becoming firm throughout the experience. Nipples are as sensitive in men as they are in women and plenty of men like theirs stimulated during lovemaking.

TEETH

Western tastes may demand that white, even teeth are the order of the day, but up until very recently Chinese women would complement their white make-up and red lipstick with blackened teeth. The Yapese, who inhabit an island in the Carolines, also believe black teeth are sexy and native Australians and many African societies think filing, decorating and pulling teeth improves a woman's or a man's sexual looks.

SKIN DEEP?

In Tonga, light, smooth skin is thought so attractive that girls will sit on cushions to keep their thighs and buttocks soft and smooth. The daughter of a chief will be bathed and oiled every evening, and when she sleeps, lies on her side with her knees tied together. This is supposed to keep her elbows smooth... and her virginity intact.

Many women believe that having smooth, unblemished skin is an important beauty requirement, while other societies deliberately scar their skin and consider this to be both beautiful and sexually arousing. Cuts are made and substances and pigments are often rubbed into the wounds to produce a scar or a tattoo. The Samoans follow this custom for both sexes, while the Bala, from Zaire, admire designs that go from the breasts down to the groin on their women. In Japan, Africa, Oceania, Britain and the United States, tattoos are found particularly on men and are seen as being

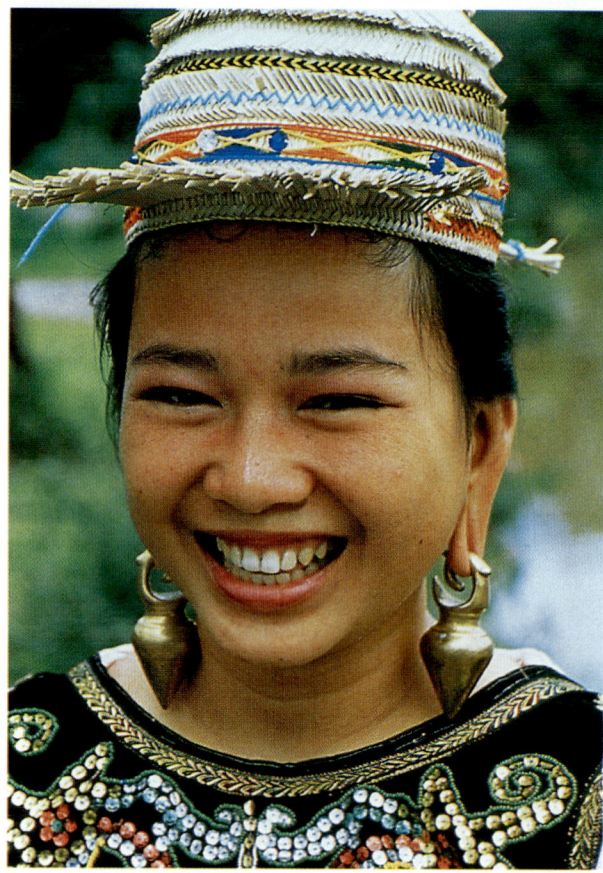

IDEAS OF BEAUTY VARY FROM CULTURE TO CULTURE. WHITE, EVEN TEETH ARE THOUGHT ATTRACTIVE IN MANY SOCIETIES, AND A SMILE IS A COME-ON WHEREVER YOU ARE

very macho. Many societies decorate the skin in less permanent ways. In ancient Egypt and China and in India today, body make-up as well as facial make-up is considered particularly attractive. In the West, women may highlight facial features and paint finger- and toenails. In India, women's hands and feet are often completely covered with elaborate painted designs.

The skin has more nerve endings than any other part of the body, constantly supplying the brain with information about the body's surroundings. Nobody, but nobody, has a bigger organ than this – about 17 square feet, or 1.6 square metres, of sensation just waiting to be used. What's more, it comes complete with its own turn-on. Where our love-life is concerned, most of us tend to think of skin only in terms of touch, but a bigger appeal could be to our sense of smell. Sweat may not seem to be much of a come-on, but mixed in with the one and a half pints that the average body produces each day is a chemical called pheromone, which sends out extremely sexy signals. Why not try Nature's way of attracting your lover? Stay fresh, but leave all the deodorants, talcum powders and perfumes alone for a while. You will probably find that the smell of the real you has far more sex appeal than anything you can get out of a bottle.

YOUR SKIN HAS A VERY SPECIAL APPEAL – AND THIS ISN'T JUST TO DO WITH HOW IT FEELS. SWEAT, ESPECIALLY FROM THE GLANDS AROUND THE GENITAL AREA, CONTAINS CHEMICALS CALLED PHEROMONES THAT ARE A REAL TURN-ON FOR SEXUAL PARTNERS

GENITALS

As to the genitals themselves, these are seen by many women to be deformed or at least unusual if the vagina is not loose enough to take a tampon or penis easily but tight and snug enough to hold it firmly. Labia can be a source of enormous anxiety to Western women, if they are perceived as being too big, too wrinkled, or hanging down too low. Many women can only remember their vulva from childhood – the neat and tidy structure with two plump cushions on either side of a slit. But the adult version is far more complex and the labia will have grown during puberty. During sexual excitement, they will expand temporarily to two, three or even four times their normal size. To allow for this, they appear wrinkled and grainy, like a balloon that has been blown up and then allowed to collapse, when they are in their relaxed

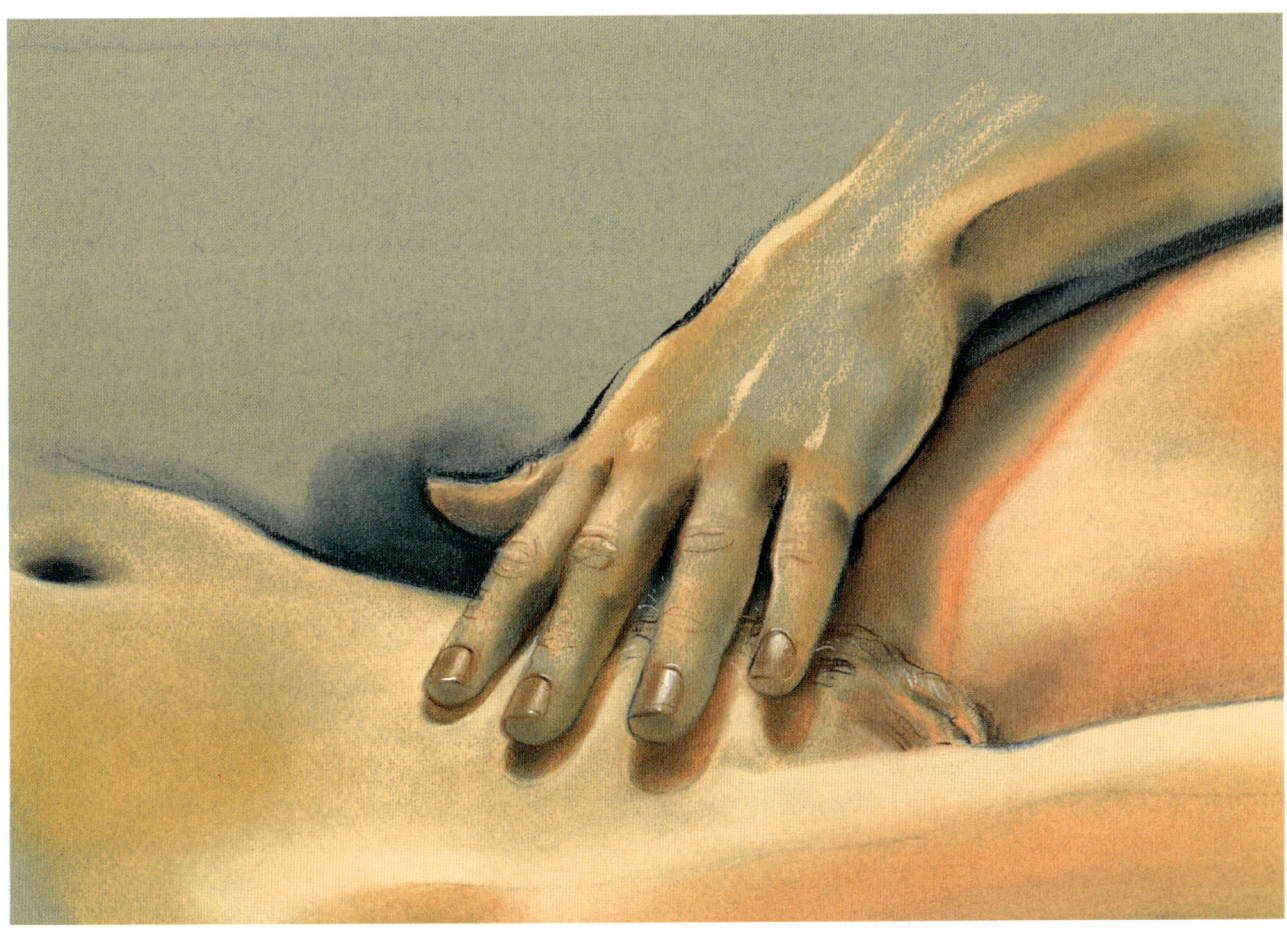

state. Also, scent and oil glands exude a rich mixture to send out signals to the opposite sex and to keep the expandable surfaces flexible. Far from seeing it as being ugly or smelly, any partner would be likely to find the appearance, scents and texture of a woman's vulva extremely exciting.

During puberty, height and weight is gained, with extra muscle and padding on her hips and his shoulders, and breasts and genitals hang out and develop, increasing in dimension and acquiring texture, taste, smell and a protective covering of hair. All this activity is often accompanied by a heightened sensitivity as these new toys cry out to be handled and tested. Sadly, most children in the West are made to feel from a very early age that self-exploration and self-pleasuring is a disgusting habit. Few get the right sort of information and so puberty may be the beginning of fear or dissatisfaction with our bodies that can last for a lifetime. The Masai, the Nyaturu and the Fipa of Tanzania have a very different approach. Not only do parents anxiously watch for signs of erection in their children's sex organs, they also positively encourage exploration. The Chaga of Tanzania even consider seeing a doctor if it doesn't occur.

Few Western children receive proper instruction about what to expect and why at puberty, and so many young people start a lifetime's habit of not coming to terms with their bodies. A masturbating girl, for example, will find touching herself makes her breasts and genitals swell, and can become convinced that the permanent changes in the appearance of her breasts and genitals taking place at this time are somehow visible proof of her "filthy habits". She may believe that the smelly, hairy and wrinkled genitals she now has must be a deformity that she must hide or somehow have altered. Perhaps she will never succeed in shaking off the fear, possibly induced by a slapped hand when she tried a little self-exploration many years previously, that somehow her body is unacceptable.

Societies that value sexual expression have a different attitude to the labia. The Tswana of Botswana and the Thonga from Mozambique consider prominent inner genital lips a major source of sexual attraction. At the onset of puberty, when the labia begin to enlarge, girls will manipulate and pull at them in an attempt to make sure theirs become long and curtain-like.

On Mangaia, in the Pacific, girls will concentrate on lengthening their clitori by manipulation, and are taught how to achieve orgasm by the women of the group. The Ila, from Zambia, also believe that women should have navels that stick out to be truly sexually attractive.

THE VAGINA

Many cultures, such as those in Zambia and in the Pacific, believe that a tight vagina is attractive and value it in a woman. To encourage this, astringents such as alum or salt or herbal poultices are often put in the sex passage, sometimes when a girl reaches puberty and sometimes in babyhood. Sadly, Western women are often persuaded that this part of the body is smelly and unclean and deodorants are used in the same spirit – to change and "clean up" the area. The effects of both of these approaches can be harmful. The vagina is self-cleansing and its tissue is fragile. Scents, soaps, deodorants, herbs and astringents can all lead to infection and damage. A simple rule is – don't put anything into your vagina that you wouldn't put in your mouth!

THE CLITORIS

The clitoris is probably the most sensitive area of a woman's body. There is a belief that women are capable of experiencing greater pleasure in sexual intercourse than men and the structure of the clitoris could support this. The sensitive clitoris contains a net of nerve endings three times as large as that of the penis in proportion to its size. While the average penis enlarges by around 50% during sexual stimulation, the average clitoris enlarges by

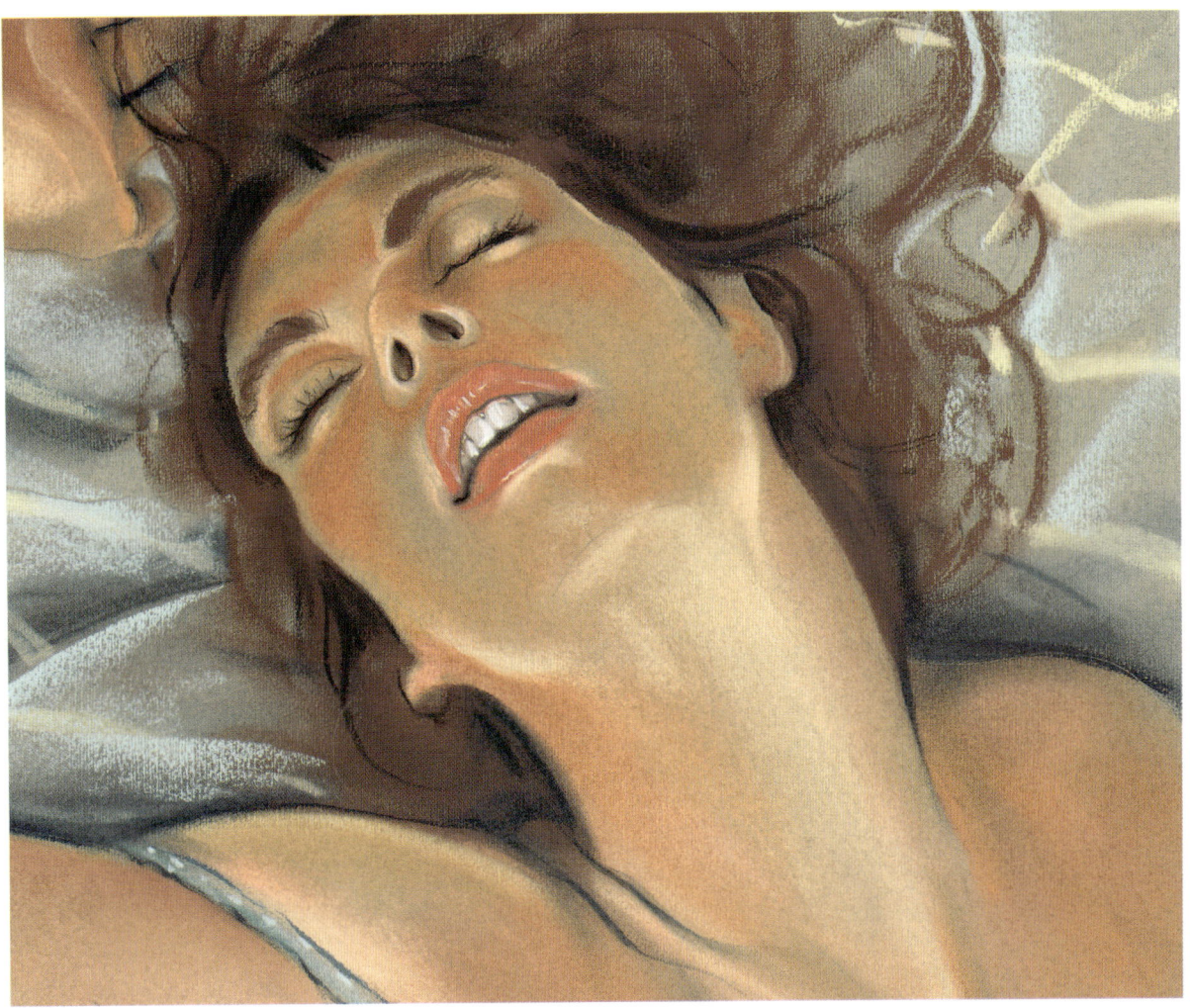

SOME SOCIETIES TEACH PEOPLE HOW TO ACHIEVE ORGASM, AND THERE ARE NOW "ORGASM WORKSHOPS" IN THE WEST

as much as two- to three-fold, although some women experience engorgement without an increase in size.

BODY HAIR

Another pet hate for many women is body hair. They see anything more than a small, neat triangle over the genitals as unfeminine, alarming and needing instant removal. Zulu women and men share this belief and remove all pubic and armpit hair by plucking and shaving. In other cultures, however, hair removal serves a particular ritual purpose. In Zambia, the Ila people expect a new bride to pluck out the hair on the face and genitals of her husband the day after consummating their marriage.

In Turkey and the Middle East, women de-fuzz their entire bodies using a boiled mixture of sugar and lemon juice and men remove the hair in their armpits. The Anglo-American style of removing hair under the armpits, on the legs and around the bikini line is catching on through much of the world. However, many women in Germany and Scandinavia – and their men – still don't believe that body hair is anything to be ashamed of and much Japanese erotica pays particular attention to men and women with outrageously hirsute (and large) genitals.

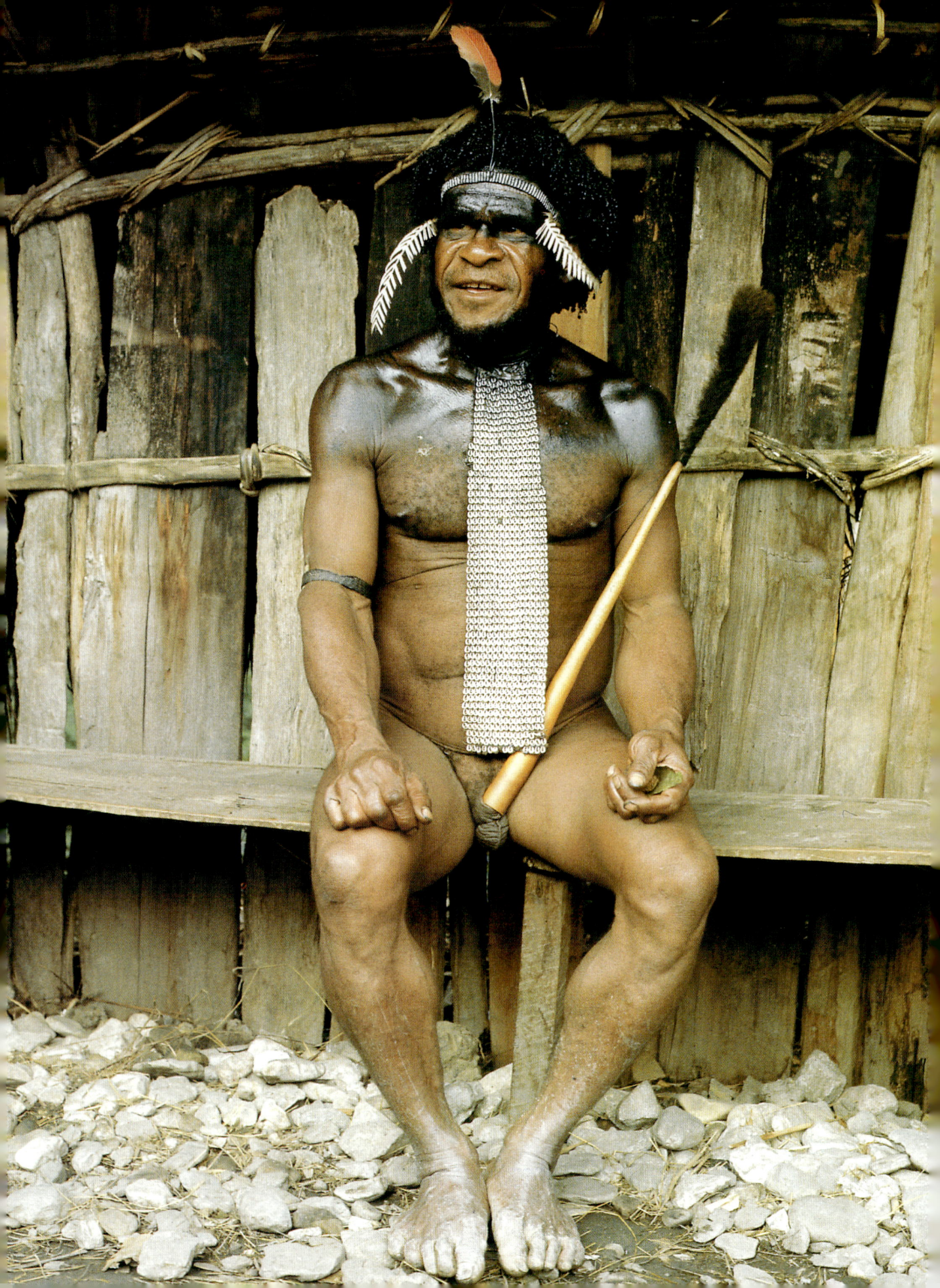

PRIVATE FEARS

It may seem that it is only women who continually worry about what they have or haven't got in the body stakes, but men too have their anxieties. They may worry that their chests are not hairy enough, or that they have missed out in the muscles stakes. But these worries are small beer compared with male worries over the mighty penis itself. Is it big enough, is the sight of it a passion- or a giggle-arouser, is it curved or is it out of the ordinary? There is also the endless debate over foreskin or circumcision. And, above all, the never-ending concern over whether the beast will perform its duties when required.

A lot of women's problems over their genitals spring from the fact that they cannot see them properly without the use of a mirror or being rubber-jointed. Men's problems, on the other hand, are largely due to being able to see their own and other men's equipment far too frequently and easily and making too many, often inaccurate, comparisons. Most of these worries could be removed if every little boy could be taught that a cylindrical object always appears longer and bigger when viewed from the side than when seen from above. This would save them from the unnecessary agony they feel when they compare their penis with another by looking down on their own, severely foreshortened member and then across at the competition. In Southern China, Malaysia and Borneo there is even a sexual disorder called *Koro*. This is an obsessive fear that the penis is shrinking and will disappear up into the stomach, with fatal results. It can be a form of mass hysteria and men afflicted with this disorder tie a cord around their penis, put it in a wooden splint or demand that members of the family take turns keeping a tight grip on the organ to prevent it disappearing. The probable cause of this strange affliction is guilt over masturbation in societies where sexual exploration is not encouraged.

Little boys should also be taught that, although male organs can differ quite dramatically when flaccid, most erect to around the same size – about 17 cm or 6½ inches. A thicker, longer penis is likely to expand far less than a thinner and shorter cousin.

Men around the world boast and show off to each other and compare penis size or strength. In many societies, men wear nothing but a penis sheath. Leaves, shells, leather and ivory have all been used to make penis sheaths. More recently, groups in South Africa and New Guinea have adapted modern materials, using toothpaste tubes and Coca Cola cans. In Norway, men take part in penis weightlifting contests, suspending pails with different amounts of water in them from erections.

Saving yourself

Among the Abkhasians, living in the Caucasus, you don't have to be young and beautiful to be thought sexually attractive. In fact, the Abkhasians, who don't believe in "dirty old men" – or women – think that saving yourself until quite late in life is far better for you. Many live to a hundred and enjoy a sexually active old age.

HEADS YOU WIN

Some societies consider the shape of the head to be particularly important when it comes to looking sexy. In certain parts of France during the early part of this century, and still among Native Americans on the north-western coast of the USA, babies' heads are moulded while the bones are still soft. Infants are bound to a board with a second board pressing on their foreheads. This flattens and pushes back the head to a point, giving it what is considered to be an attractive outline.

SOME MEN ARE ONLY TOO WILLING TO SHOW OFF THE TRADITIONAL MALE PRIDE IN THE PENIS!

STICKING YOUR NECK OUT

The most trusting movement an animal can make – and humans are animals too! – is to expose the throat. Lying head-back and relaxed is a sign of love and security, which is often recognized unconsciously as proof of complete confidence in your companion. The Japanese are in no doubt of the erotic potential of the neck. The nape of the neck is one of the few parts of the body that their women have always left exposed, even in their otherwise all-concealing national costume. In Burma, among the Padaung, women are thought attractive only if they have long, slender necks. Ring after ring is placed around the women's necks until they stretch to twice their normal length.

EARS

When it comes to the sexual potential of ears, Jolan Chang, in his *The Tao of Love and Sex*, says that "For men, the most sensitive area apart from the phallus is the inside of the ear." Perhaps we do unconsciously still recognize the ear's appeal. It is significant that earrings are increasingly popular, with both sexes, and that piercing ears is one of the few "tribal" physical mutilations still used in Western society.

THE NECK IS MUCH MORE OF AN EROGENOUS ZONE THAN YOU MIGHT THINK. STROKING, NIBBLING, LICKING AND KISSING YOUR PARTNER HERE MAY HAVE A STRIKING EFFECT – SO WHY NOT TRY IT OUT?

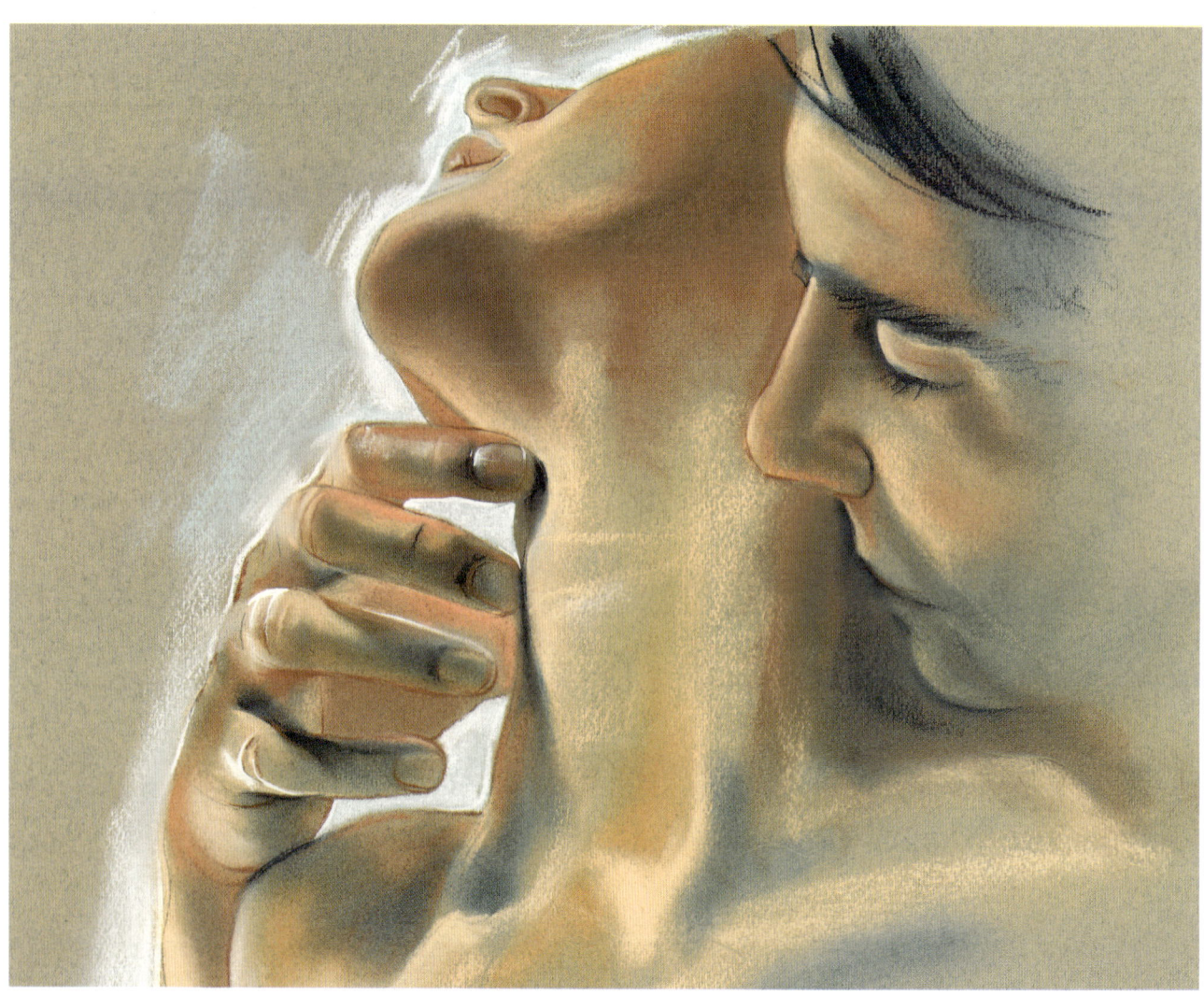

The ear is full of nerves and blood vessels and is very sensitive. There are approximately 50 acupuncture points in each ear where needles may be placed with effect, and "auriculotherapists" claim the ears can influence the whole body if they are gently massaged, pulled or pinched. The middle and inner ear are very delicate and extremely sensitive to pressure changes. Blow gently, and stroke, don't poke. The only things you should put in your loved one's ear are an exploring tongue or sweet words.

Extreme sexual excitement, and even orgasm, can be obtained from skilful stroking, blowing or sucking on and around the ear and neck. Sadly, many people in the West still associate blowing in the ears or planting vampire-like love bites on the neck with the first sexual fumbles of acned youth, or scenes from early movies. Yet, if the claims of various therapists are to be believed, we are wasting our natural resources in underusing these erogenous zones.

NUDITY

Obviously, clothing does have its practical purposes – if the temperature is below freezing it's not just modesty that suggests we cover up. But how we wear clothes often has as much to do with emphasizing or concealing parts of the body as protecting ourselves from the elements. In some Muslim societies, women are required to cover their faces and sometimes their entire bodies. One explanation would be that this protects them from the unwelcome attention of men, another that it protects men from the unwelcome distraction of female beauty. An alternative explanation would be that it keeps women subservient. In Chad, some women also wear veils, but these are elaborate, beaded affairs – and it's the only clothing they wear. Among the Tuareg of the Sahara, veils are worn only by men.

Complete nakedness is actually fairly rare among human societies. In the Sudan, men of the Dinka go totally naked, as do Brazilian women of the Mundurucu, but in most other societies something is used, if only beads or penis sheaths as a decoration. This means that since clothing conceals, taking it off can make certain statements. We are all familiar with the idea of the artful and enticing striptease. Among some social groups, however, bearing parts of the body can have a very different meaning. In a practice called *whackapohane*, Maoris show contempt for people, or make political protest, by exposing their buttocks.

In the West, it's often felt that revealing acres of skin is an invitation to have sex. Not so with many other peoples – the Zulu of South Africa consider clothing to be a way of covering up immorality rather than the other way round. The Tonga of the South Pacific have a ritual in which a high-status girl who is a virgin will dance naked. Rather than being seen as erotic, this is accepted as a way of actually openly proclaiming her chastity.

However, nudity is catching on more and more in the West, particularly at the beach, and isn't necessarily seen as an invitation to sex – or at least, it isn't in the societies in which this behaviour is common. In places such as Turkey, Greece and the North African coast, showing skin is kept to very private behaviour and so women who go topless may receive very unwelcome attention from residents.

So you can see that what each of us finds sexy can differ surprisingly from one culture to another. But surely we are all the same, under the skin? Love and marriage seem to be the principal aims of most men and women... aren't they? In fact, there is an enormous diversity in the nature of love, the rituals of courtship, the function of marriage and the manner of sex throughout the world, and we will look much more closely at some of these fascinating variations in the next chapter.

Love, Courtship & Marriage

It doesn't matter which country you come from, love, courtship, sex and marriage will be present in some form in your life. But the actual form that these important life stages take can vary to a surprising extent around the world.

In some cultures, marriage is a private contract, based on romantic love. In various other groups, it is a social arrangement meant to benefit the community rather than the individuals concerned. Partners may be assigned to each other by their family or by leaders of their community, and marriages might even be conducted en masse, as shown here

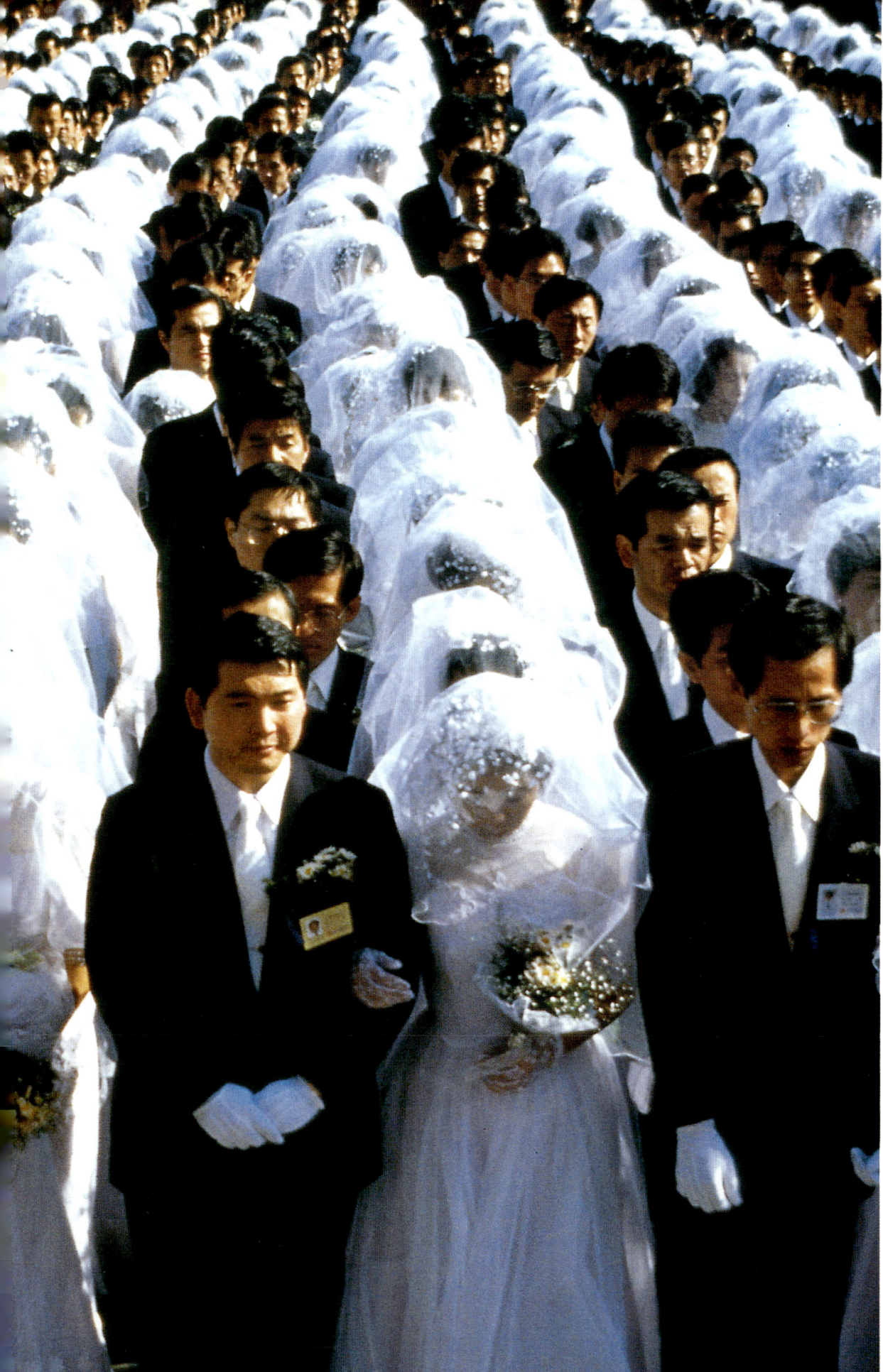

Talking about it, learning about it

And before we even get to the age when we want to start sexual activity, we learn the ropes from our "elders and betters". In some societies, this means active instruction from relatives; in some it is classroom lessons. In others, it means the unspoken understanding that you don't ever talk about the subject.

In some communities, what parents pass on is very upfront. As we heard in Chapter 1, various groups in Tanzania constantly check their babies' sex organs to see if they erect when they are being fed or cuddled and will sometimes help them to do so. Children are encouraged to touch themselves and hear about sex as an integral part of their instruction in being good citizens and good husbands and wives.

Practice makes perfect

Boys of the Gogo in Tanzania learn how to masturbate in a very fruity way. Older boys will suggest they take a watermelon, bore a hole in it and discover the joys of sex in that way.

Coming-of-age

All societies see the transition between childhood and adulthood as a vital time of your life. Not only are young people expected to learn about themselves and their place in the community, they are often also expected to take part in important rituals to mark this journey from child to grown-up. Among the Ila of Zambia, boys have to learn how to masturbate and ape sexual intercourse with each other as part of their initiation training. In several African societies, boys have sex with a married woman as part of their initiation ceremony. In Western society, coming of age rituals mean a party and gifts. For Nigerians, a first period is the signal for a great feast, to welcome a girl into adulthood.

Mother and son

Among the Tukanao, Native Americans of Brazil, boys undergo a coming-of-age initiation ritual that includes having sexual intercourse with their mother in the presence of their father.

Rites of passage

What made you feel you were an adult, rather than a child? Was it a party, a present or something your parents did for you? Or was it something you and your friends did in secret, like smoking a first cigarette, having sex, driving a car...? Perhaps something happened to you that took you by surprise, such as a first period or wet dream, and maybe you felt you couldn't talk about it. Was it a positive experience, with everyone around you in favour of you and what you were doing? Or was it a mixed blessing, and something risky that was done in defiance of the adult world?

Looking at the way other cultures manage this transition between childhood and adulthood, do you think your group did it as well, better or worse? Think about whether the way you passed from one stage of your life to another might have affected the way you manage your love-life and relationships. And, crazy as it sounds, if you don't think you were given a good enough welcome to adulthood then, do it for yourself now!

Some societies openly accept that learning about sex may involve practical lessons

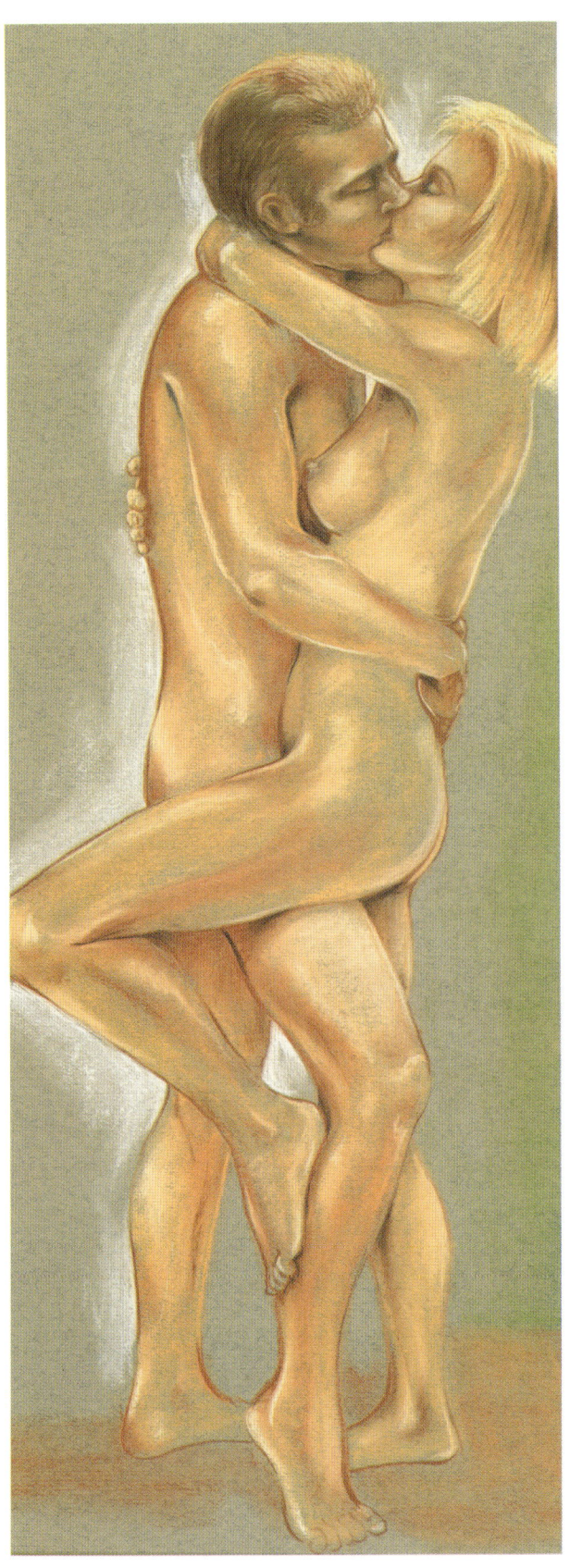

In some cultures, such as the Masai in Kenya, learning about your body and about relationships isn't just a case of talking about it or practising with friends of the same sex. From the age of seven, boys and girls are allowed to sleep together and to experiment with sex play and even intercourse. Masai men and women are expected to be faithful after marriage, but being a virgin bride is so unimportant that there isn't even a word in their language for virgin! Competence in lovemaking is seen to be a desirable quality in both a wife and a husband.

These beliefs are also common in other parts of Africa. Among the Ngoni, if a girl doesn't take a lover after puberty, her grandmother will worry so much that the girl is not able to be sexual that she will actually go out, find a young man, and get the two together. He will be rewarded for discovering whether the girl is sexually "normal".

In Britain and the United States, encouraging young people to have sex before marriage would horrify many adults. In spite of the fact that the majority of people do have their first sexual experience before getting married, lip service is still paid to the idea that it is naughty. Good sex education programmes often founder on the fear that talking about sex to young people encourages them to "do it". Studies don't bear this out, and young people who are encouraged to be open about sex are usually found to start their sex lives later than those who are deprived of frank information.

In the Netherlands, teenagers get pregnant twelve times less often than in North America and seven times less often than in Britain. What's more, they tend to start their sex lives slightly later. Yet, young people in the Netherlands get considerably more sex education than teenagers in Britain or the States. There are sexually explicit television and radio programmes on at all times, and sex educators tour the holiday resorts in summer, handing out condoms and advice. In Sweden, the picture is the same. During the winter, representatives of the Swedish family planning association, RFSU, patrol the ski slopes offering free contraceptive supplies. In summer, they take their "Love Bus" to the beach, offering advice, condoms and stick-on, temporary tattoos with safer sex messages.

In Thailand, the entire sex education and family planning scene was transformed under the pioneering influence of one man, Mechai Viravaidya. He took his highly entertaining sex education "roadshow" around villages in an attempt to make sex and contraception subjects that people of all ages could talk about. Thailand even has "The Family Planning Buffalo"! Families who are using contraception, where husband or wife have been sterilized for instance, can hire a buffalo at cheap rates to till their fields, a concession not available to those who are not planning their families responsibly.

Of course, the things you hear from your elders and betters are not always helpful. In Catholic Latin America, young girls tend to be given very negative messages about sex and men while they are single. As soon as they get married, of course, they are supposed to be loving and sexy with their husbands – a difficult transition to make. Every culture has folk beliefs about sex that are wildly inaccurate. For instance, many teenagers in various different cultures believe you can't get pregnant if you have sex standing up or if the woman doesn't have an orgasm.

Why do different cultures have such opposing approaches? When Paul the Apostle put the fear of God into the Romans with his message that "the wages of sin is death", there was no doubt in his mind that the mortal body was the cause of all human ills. Paul may only have been trying to put one small group of early Christians on the straight and narrow, but the belief that sex is dirty and brings fear and punishment is still an important factor in many Western and Christian cultures today.

In Old Testament times, the main distinction between what was good and what was sinful was based on the practical need to be procreative. Any sexual act that didn't have this end in view was condemned, and this view has lingered on – Western cultures still consider masturbation and homosexual sex to be wrong. In various non-Western societies, non-reproductive sex, and sex outside child-bearing partnerships, is seen in a different way. In many societies, the deciding factor is how to keep women and their childbearing potential as a man's possession. Doing this maintains a certain kind of status quo, a predictable sense of order. It is a particular society's view of what constitutes orderliness that dictates what is acceptable in different cultures. So, in yet another cultural style, sex is seen as a gift from the gods, to be enjoyed and celebrated. Or simply, as a normal part of life that needs to be understood and practised, like any other skill.

Talking about it

Can you talk about sex to your partner? If not, why not? Is it because of the way you learned about sex when you were young? Think about the way you heard about sexual matters. Is your background more like the British – stiff upper lip (but nothing else!) and don't talk about the dirty stuff? Or is it more like the Dutch – lots of information and discussion? Or is it like the Masai – talk, encouragement and hands-on practice? Work out with your partner the way you might have liked to have learned about sex, and then go out and make up for it now – it's never too late to learn.

THE DATING GAME

"Courting" rituals of one kind or another are found all over the world. But how exactly men and women show their interest in each other varies across the continents.

In Papua New Guinea, if a man wants to pay court to a woman, he takes a hair from his head, one from his shoulders and one from his groin and rolls them into a cigarette. He then smokes half and gives the other half to his mother, who gives it to the woman he has chosen. If she smokes it she is accepting his proposal of marriage.

PREMARITAL SEX

The Sukuma of Tanzania say they disapprove of premarital sex. However, they have a traditional game that positively encourages it, called *chagulaga mayu*. After dances, girls are surrounded by admiring men who go up to girls they fancy and say *chagulaga*, which means "choose the one you love". A girl then goes up to the boy she wants, touches him and runs off. He pursues her and if he can't catch her is jeered at by everyone. If he does catch her, he's allowed to pull her into the bushes, where the couple can go as far as they like. Premarital pregnancy means disgrace for the girl and a fine in cattle for the boy, but the game still goes on. This is because the game can be a good way for couples to see if they could be fertile together and it often ends up in marriage.

Similarly, premarital sex among the West African Ashanti may be seen as a form of courting and is called *mpena awaree* or "lover marriage". In practice, most couples have a *mpena awaree* before going on to a formal marriage. In much of Western society today, courting behaviour is basically very similar. The majority of brides and grooms lose their virginity before getting married, but in many cases have only had sex with the partner they then marry.

As you can see, in some societies, such as in Tanzania, the elders of the group consider that how to court, how to romance and even how to have sex are important parts of the education that all teenagers should be given. What happens in other societies?

In many European and Western groups, teenagers pick up these skills in an informal way. They fumble along the best they can, learning by watching, listening and trial and error. You often learn best by having role models – older people you love and admire to show you the way. In societies where families are large, or where people of all ages tend to go to social gatherings together, young people pick up social skills from older brothers and sisters, young aunts and uncles or neighbours. But in most industrial countries, families are now smaller and people tend to go out just with their own age group. This often means that you don't have anyone to watch who is a few years ahead of you in the dating game. Perhaps this is why some people feel that Western teenagers are losing their ability to charm, chat up and ask out potential partners. In Italy today, once felt by non-Italians and the Italians themselves to be the home of romance, some enterprising social experts have noticed this problem and are offering courses to help both men and women learn and practise the art of charm and enticement.

One form of courting behaviour found in societies as far apart as Polynesia and the Philippines, North and South America, is "night crawling". This is a sexual practice in which young men, and sometimes young women, creep through the night into their neighbours' huts and climb into bed with a partner they fancy. Sometimes, kissing and fondling is all that goes on, but at other times it can be full sexual intercourse.

Night crawling is easy in countries with hot climates, where families tend to sleep in communal groups in large, open houses. Another form of night courting is found in cultures that live in cold climates. This is called "bundling" and it occurs today in some remote parts of

Scandinavia. Couples are allowed to sleep together – but only if they are tightly bundled up in layers of warm clothing that are supposed to prevent any naughty stuff!

TEENAGE BRIDES AND DECEMBER WEDDINGS

The age at which you marry can be surprisingly different depending on your culture. The Zande, of the Congo-Sudan, believe in delaying marriage until men and women are in their thirties or forties. For this reason, sexual relationships between men are said to be extremely common. In Nigeria, the Igbo expect a husband-to-be to give a large payment to his in-laws, reimbursing them for raising their daughter and proving that he's responsible enough to become a married man. It can take quite a few years to raise the necessary wedding capital, and so Igbo men tend to marry late. In contrast, child marriage and betrothal is still found in some parts of the world. On Melville, an Australasian island, Tiwi families betroth their children before they are even conceived, as do the Yanomamo of South America and the Zande of Africa. The Kadar of Nigeria marry off their daughters by the time they are six years old, although this doesn't necessarily mean children have sex at a very early age.

WHY DO PEOPLE MARRY?

In the West, people choose their own partners, and marry for love. In practice, men and women tend to fall for people their families get along with, but even if they don't, the choice is understood to be an individual one. In many cultures, however,

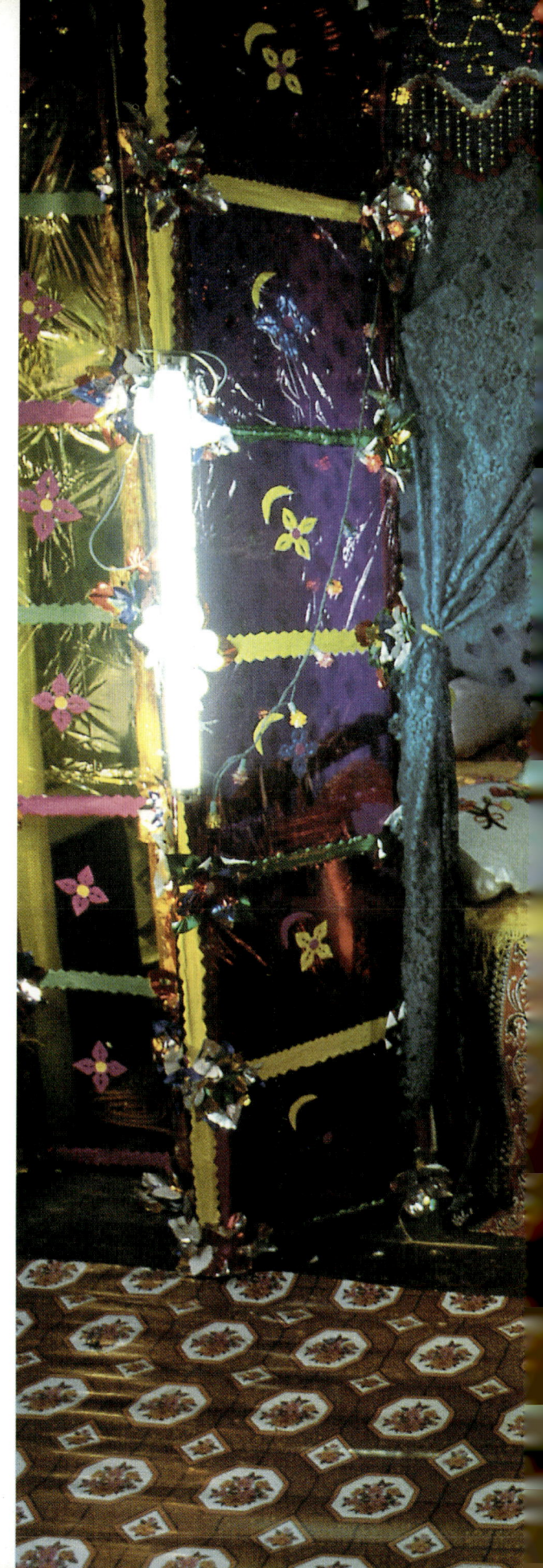

TEENAGE BRIDES, SUCH AS THE GIRL SHOWN HERE, ARE THE NORM IN SOME SOCIETIES, WITH TWENTY-SOMETHINGS CONSIDERED PAST THEIR BEST! THE WEST STILL HAS ITS FAIR SHARE OF TEENAGE BRIDES, WHO OFTEN MARRY BECAUSE A BABY IS ON THE WAY. HOWEVER, THE AVERAGE AGE FOR FIRST MARRIAGE IN THE WEST IS MID- TO LATE TWENTIES.

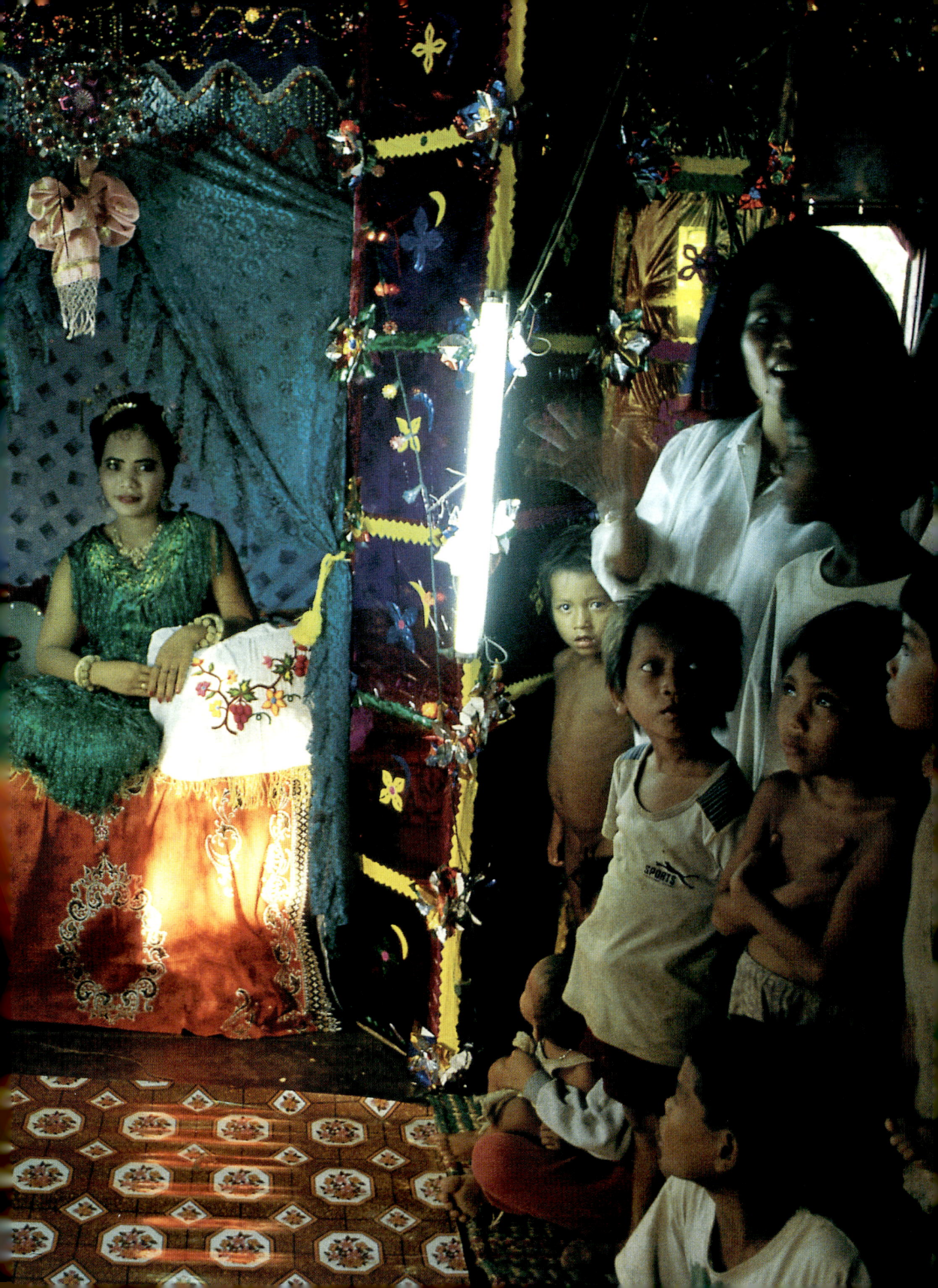

marriage is more of a social arrangement, something that is undertaken principally for the good of the community.

Marriages are arranged in most of the Islamic world – in Africa, South-east Asia, India and Japan. Fathers, mothers or a professional matchmaker will enquire around the community to find a suitable partner. In some parts of Asia, couples are brought together before a betrothal and have an opportunity to get to know each other, even if it's only for one meeting in the presence of the rest of the family. Sometimes, if the bride or groom to be really takes against their intended, the marriage will be called off. But in some groups, the first time they meet may be at the ceremony itself, and personal likes and dislikes are totally irrelevant. This is because marriage is not felt to be about private feelings, but about having children and continuing the family line.

In Japan, Korea, Taiwan, Thailand and Hawaii, the institution of marriage is an important part of society but provides little comfort for the wife. Men put far more energy into their work and their friendships with other men than into family life. Time off work is generally spent in bars and they seek erotic satisfaction with prostitutes and hostesses, or mistresses if they can afford them. Instead of a loving relationship, the wife has her home, her children and a television to keep her company.

The marriage trap

In Andalusia in Spain, men believe women only want to trap them in marriage to have children, and that once the children are grown, the women would rather dispose of the men and live on their insurance. Andalusian women are all thought to be sex-mad and the men spend a lot of their time trying to abstain from sexual intercourse, convinced that women go out of their way to drain men of their vitality and to drive them into an early grave by demanding sex. Men in Andalusia are so certain that all women would be unfaithful, given the opportunity, that it's considered bad manners to say a baby looks like its mother. This would beg the obvious question, does it or does it not resemble its supposed father?

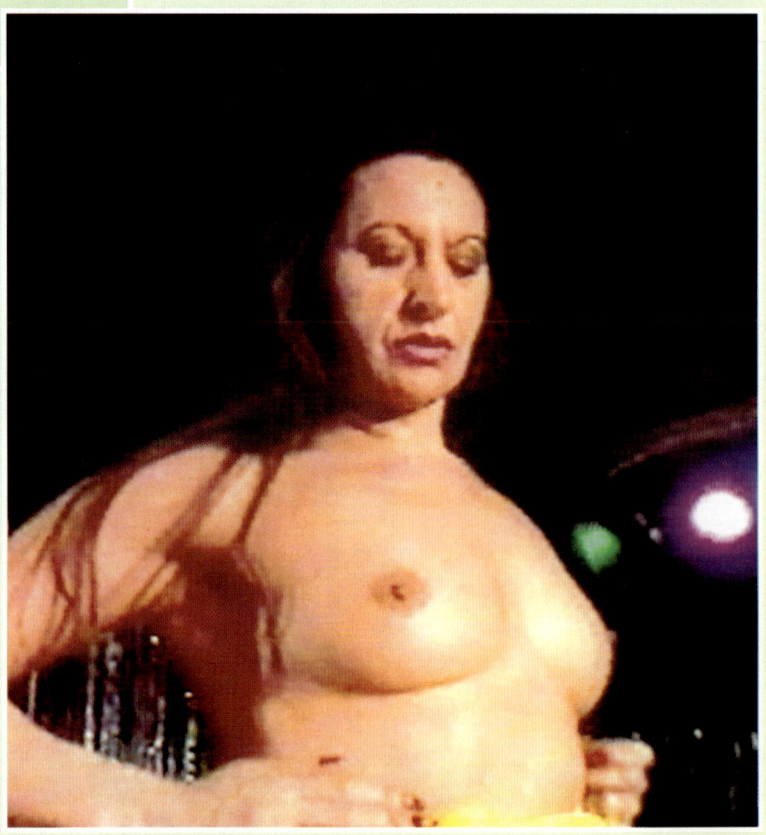

FOR THIS SPANISH WOMAN, SEX IS AN ADDICTION. WHETHER ADDICTS CRAVE ORGASM OR THE ILLUSION OF LOVE AND ATTENTION IS A MATTER FOR DEBATE

Ashanti marriages tend to be simple and private, with no particular celebration. Marriage among the Ashanti does not seem to make for much personal happiness in itself. Brides continue to live with their parents and their husbands pay them very little attention. They will visit their wives for sex, but eat and sleep at their own houses. In fact, the only way an Ashanti wife can measure her husband's regard for her is by the amount of housekeeping money that he gives her.

The Naayar of India are another group in which marriage may not have the same meaning as it does for Westerners. Before a girl starts her periods, the Naayar will hold a lengthy ceremony for her that lasts for four days. The girl is linked to a man who becomes her ritual husband. But far from settling down with him, this "marriage" frees her to have as many visiting husbands as she likes. She goes on living in her mother's home and her lovers will spend the night but not move in with her. If a Naayar gets pregnant when she hasn't been through this ceremony, she is disgraced and her children seen as illegitimate; if it is after the ceremony, they are considered to be legitimate.

A marriage for pleasure

Among some Muslims and Shi'as in Iran and parts of Iraq, temporary marriage is still accepted. Mikah al-mut'a is a "marriage for pleasure" and it can be celebrated for a night or several days. A dowry may change hands and, if the woman becomes pregnant, the child is legitimate, but neither the child nor the mother have any claim on the father.

However, in many societies, marriage is seen to be a most desirable state for both men and women. Among the Tanzanian Fipa, marriage is prized and celebrated. Both husbands and wives are expected to please each other in bed and while she wears beads and ornaments to be attractive, to be a good husband he must be knowledgeable in the arts of love. In the West, marriage is thought to be good for you and the best social arrangement for an adult to have. Although unmarried men are often thought to have the most fun, studies suggest the opposite. A German survey found that faithful, sexually satisfied husbands were far more effective at work than either single men or husbands who were having affairs.

Back to nature

The Sarakatsani of Greece feel it is such a disgrace to die unmarried that spinsters or bachelors are buried in wedding clothes so as to transform the funeral into a wedding to Mother Nature.

WHO'S ELIGIBLE?

Some societies are pretty free and easy about who you can marry, but in others the rules are so strict that it can really narrow down your options. For instance, the Mende of West Africa and the Copts of Egypt think that incest doesn't just occur between people with the same parents. The Koran forbids marriage, not only between blood relatives but also between "milk relatives". "Milk incest" occurs between anyone who has been breastfed by the same woman. Italian Roman Catholics and Eastern Orthodox Christians share this belief too. Since in these societies children are often fed by wet nurses, a parent has to be pretty careful when choosing a wet nurse for the sake of their child's future happiness. Among the Dard of Afghanistan, if a couple even drink milk together this makes them milk relatives and they cannot marry.

The Mehinaku of central Brazil have so many prohibitions about who you can marry that young people may find up to two thirds of the eligible partners in their social group are off-limits to them. But not all cultures totally forbid incest or the marriage of related people. The Lamet of South-east Asia permit brother and sister marriage if the couple have been brought up in different households.

Twin marriage

On Bali, and among the Aymara of South America, a twin brother and sister are allowed to marry. This is because they are believed to have already been intimate in the womb. The Marshallese of the Pacific also believe that twins have committed incest in the womb. However, they are less forgiving and will kill either both the children or just the boy at birth.

In some societies, marriage between the living and the dead is not uncommon. Those who follow ancient Chinese traditions betroth children at a young age. This means that they may both die before they are old enough to get married, in which case a ceremony is held to bring them together after their deaths. American Mormons believe marriage is a necessary precondition to being saved and going to heaven. Even a dead unbeliever may be saved by a posthumous marriage to a Mormon.

MARRIAGE RITUALS

You may have heard of the Sabine women of Ancient Rome, who were carried away by their husbands-to-be. A similar form of bride abduction happens in quite a few societies today. In some cases it is just a ritual, a sort of game which goes on after the families have actually agreed to the wedding, giving spice to the marriage ceremony. Sometimes, however, the capture is for real.

Among the Pacific Tikopia people, young men will snatch the woman of their choice and take her home. Next day a feast is held and the husband and his family will issue a proclamation of marriage. They then may force the girl to consummate the marriage in public as a way of making sure that her family won't demand her return.

The right to choose

The Siberian society of the Kamchadal have another form of bride capture. To make a marriage legal, the groom must touch his bride's naked vulva. She dresses up in layers of clothes and surrounds herself with all her friends and the other women of the village. The eager husband-to-be must fight his way through the scrum, tear off her clothes and attempt to get his hands on her. If he fails, the marriage is annulled. If he succeeds, it's celebrated. The point of this is that it allows women some say in who they marry. If she is keen on him, she and her friends will only put up a token struggle, but if she is not happy with her father's choice, they can all fight like crazy to resist the unwanted male.

POLYGAMY

Polygamy means multiple marriage – when a man has several wives or a woman has several husbands. Among the Todas of southern India, a woman will not only have several husbands, usually all brothers, but also several officially recognized lovers. Polygamous societies are found all over the world. Among the Zulus of South Africa, the Thonga in Mozambique, many Native American groups and societies in north-eastern Asia, Papua New Guinea, the New Hebrides and the Solomon Islands, a man is allowed to have several wives but they are all sisters.

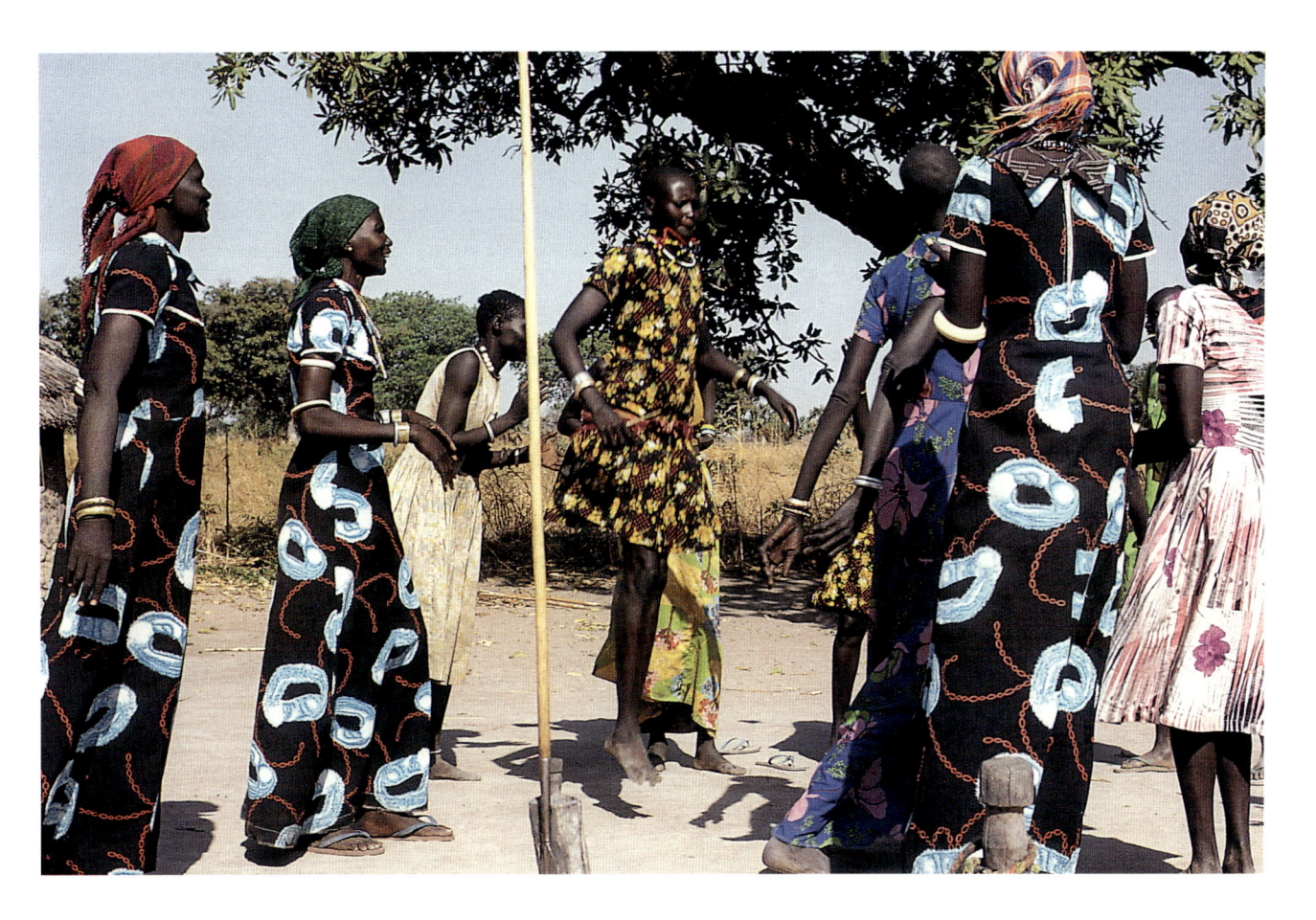

Ashanti women may have rather more than the same dressmaker in common – these women live together and share the same husband

Polygamy

In the West, the only sort of marriage accepted as correct is monogamy – one man and one woman at a time. But of 862 cultures throughout the world, only 16% insist on monogamy. It is thought to be the norm to have more than one wife at a time in 44% of cultures, while 39% consider polygamy and monogamy to be equally acceptable. The rest have a variety of arrangements.

Polygamy tends to be an indication of status and wealth. Among Samoans, for instance, only the chiefs have more than one wife. But polygamy can also be seen as an essential part of keeping families and communities going. In Ecuador, the Cayapa believe that having more than one wife is sinful – but they all do it, simply because a larger family can provide more assistance with the banana crop, their main food source.

The Pahaarii of northern India are the only known society to practise group marriage today. Custom demands that a man pay a very high price to the bride's family for his wife. Brothers will pool their resources to buy a wife in common for all of them. Various people in Europe, Australia and the US also practise a form of group marriage, creating communities where several family units live and work together, and Israel has its collective farms, or kibbutz.

In the West, one-to-one marriages are usually seen as preferable, because of the beliefs and expectations surrounding marriage. In places like Mali, the Cameroon and Senegal, women may say that they welcome having co-wives, to keep them company and help with the chores.

WEDDING DAYS, WEDDING NIGHTS

Wedding rituals can go from the practical to the bizarre. After marriage ceremonies in rural Hungary, the bride is snatched back by her family, who spirit her back to the parental home. The bridegroom gathers all his friends and

Polyandry

Westerners tend to consider polygamy as being a very male affair – they automatically think of societies where a man has several wives. But this isn't always the case, and there are cultures where women have several husbands. While polygamy is a general term used for multiple marriage, one man and two or more wives is known more specifically as polygyny and one woman with two or more husbands is called polyandry.

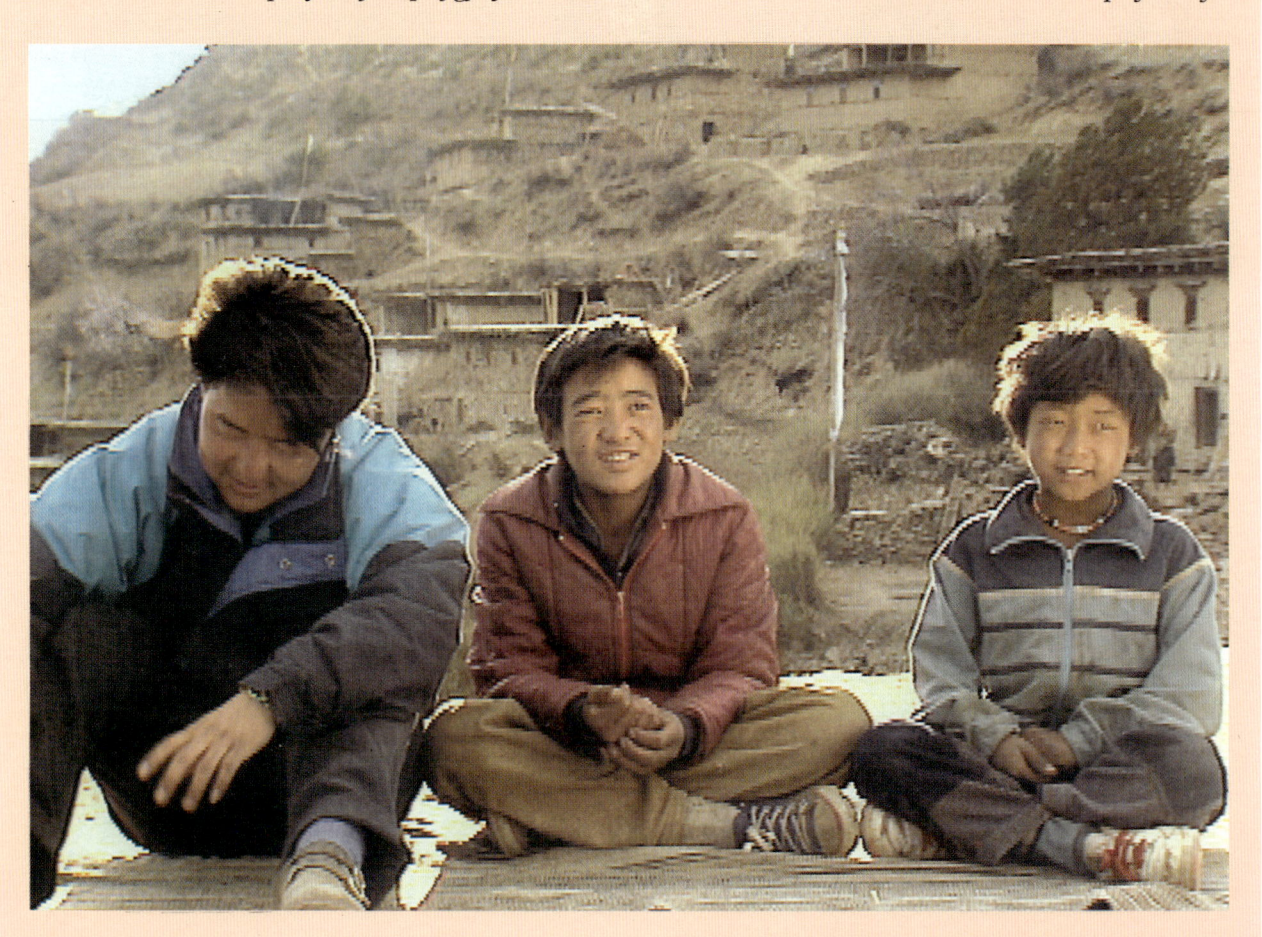

SOME SOCIETIES ARRANGE THINGS SO THAT YOUNGER BOYS WILL JOIN THEIR ELDER BROTHER IN MARRYING HIS WIFE

family and arrives at the house, where he explains that he has lost his bride and asks them to help him find her. The family bring out a succession of women, whom he rejects, until the bride emerges and the party begins.

In the British Midlands, it is thought lucky for a woman to get married wearing no underwear, and wearing "something old, something new, something borrowed, something blue" is common throughout Britain. In many societies, guests throw rice, grain or something that represents these, as a fertility blessing. At Jewish weddings, the bridegroom breaks a glass, and a dish or jar is broken in other cultures. This could be seen as a way of frightening away evil spirits, or as symbolic of the breaking of the bride's maidenhead.

In many societies, a girl's virginity is considered to be valuable and even magic. She and her family may suffer enormous shame if she is found not to be a virgin on her wedding night and sometimes a bloody sheet has to be displayed the morning after the wedding in order to prove her status. But in some Hindu, Indonesian and South American societies, infant girls as young as a month old have their maidenheads ritually stretched and broken. This is not done to save her pain or shock on her first sexual experience. It's usually done because taking a girl's virginity is believed to be so fraught with significance that a husband may be struck down with illness or some supernatural punishment if he does it. In modern Egypt, men may insist on wrapping a piece of cloth around their index finger to test their brides before going to bed with them. In some parts of Greece, it is the mother-in-law who conducts this test.

Among the Zaramo of Tanzania, the first sexual encounter on the wedding night is crucial. Zaramo women are expected to be virgins and men to be fertile and virile. So, the happy couple go to bed with two women standing over them. These spectators watch to see how easily the bride is penetrated. If she has no pain and there is no bleeding, they may decide she's had sex before the wedding night. Just before the groom comes, he will be expected to pull out and ejaculate outside his wife. The watching women will then look at the amount and the consistency of his semen. It needs to be thick and profuse for them to accept him as a real man. Nyaturu and Chaga wives, from Tanzania, are expected to resist their husbands on their wedding nights to show that they are virgins. In turn, husbands are expected to show that they have experience by insisting on their conjugal rights.

Marriage and children

In many cultures, having children is a vital part of marriage. So much so that in rural Latin America couples live together before getting married to see if they are fertile. Once a child is born, the union is made official. In the Western world, more and more couples are now living together without marrying, but with every intention of staying together. If and when a child arrives, however, some do formalize the arrangement.

Quite a few societies are reasonably tolerant of who exactly fathers children and who then brings them up. In Africa, a man of the Gwari who is impotent or infertile may allow his wife to become pregnant by another man. Any children she has are considered his even if everyone knows they were conceived with another man. Among several south Indian groups in Kerala, in the Caucasus and among some Serbians in the former Yugoslavia, there is a practice called "seed raising". A young boy will be married to an older girl or woman and until he is old enough to consummate his relationship with her, his father may have sex with her. If she has a child as a result of having sex with her father-in-law, the child will be raised as her husband's, not as her father-in-law's.

GENDER AND MARRIAGE

In Africa, women of the Kuriar, the Nuer, the Lovedu, the Dahomey Igbo and the Zulu nations, may marry other women. Although there are suggestions that these may be gay relationships, the general understanding is that it is a way for wealthy women to keep from surrendering their property (and their freedom) to a husband. They also have the opportunity to have children, since they are considered the co-parents or mothers of any children their wives have by any lover. In the USA and Europe, a similar pattern is emerging among gay couples of both sexes, who are increasingly bringing in a man or woman to give them a child. The biological parent may have no further involvement or may have visiting rights; the three might even set up home together.

LOVE IN LATER LIFE

In many parts of the world, sex really is the preserve of the young. At marriage, part of the dowry paid by a husband-to-be of the Meru of Kenya will be a large container of wood and skin filled with honey. This represents three things: the love the groom feels for his bride, the beginning of their sex life together and the ending of the sex life of her mother! In Taiwan, the Hokkien insist that both men and women stop having sex when they become grandparents. But in other societies, sex doesn't stop when the wrinkles arrive. In Florida, a part of the USA that has become the senior citizen's paradise, men and women are reclaiming sex as a proper pastime for old age. Workshops are held to relearn dating skills and to brush up on sex technique. Social occasions at which more is on offer than coffee and doughnuts are in great demand.

LOVE, MARRIAGE AND A THIRD PARTY

In Italy, France and Japan, a mistress is a socially acceptable addition to the sum – in fact, she is a sign of elegance, wealth and power. A husband is thought to be "faithful" if he treats his wife with respect and makes sure his extra-marital activities stay discreet. But, in all of these societies, what is sauce for the gander is certainly not sauce for the goose. Women are expected to be faithful to their husbands and if they are not, pay a terrible social penalty. In parts of the Middle East, men may divorce their wives, not only for infidelity or even the suspicion of it, but simply because they choose to do so. Women may not divorce men.

In the Christian West, we tend to see civilization as being the product of a struggle to subdue our sexuality. However, in the Middle East, they see true civilization to be the product of satisfied sexuality. Muslims particularly consider sexual pleasure on Earth to be just a foretaste of the pleasures of paradise to come. How we actually enjoy sex and the techniques we employ to obtain that enjoyment are many and various. We shall be considering a wide range in the next chapter.

LOVE NEED NOT FADE AS HAIR TURNS GREY, AND THIS APPLIES TO A HEALTHY INTEREST IN GOOD SEX, TOO

Sex for seniors

Many societies see old age as being non-sexual, particularly for women. The idea seems to be that once pregnancy is no longer a possibility, sex goes out the window. But we have sex for many reasons other than having children, and these don't change as the years pass. Better health, increased fitness and longer lifespans now mean we can spend up to half of our lives in the post-childbearing age group, so why should sex only be for the other half? It's healthy, fun and the best way of keeping a spring in your step.

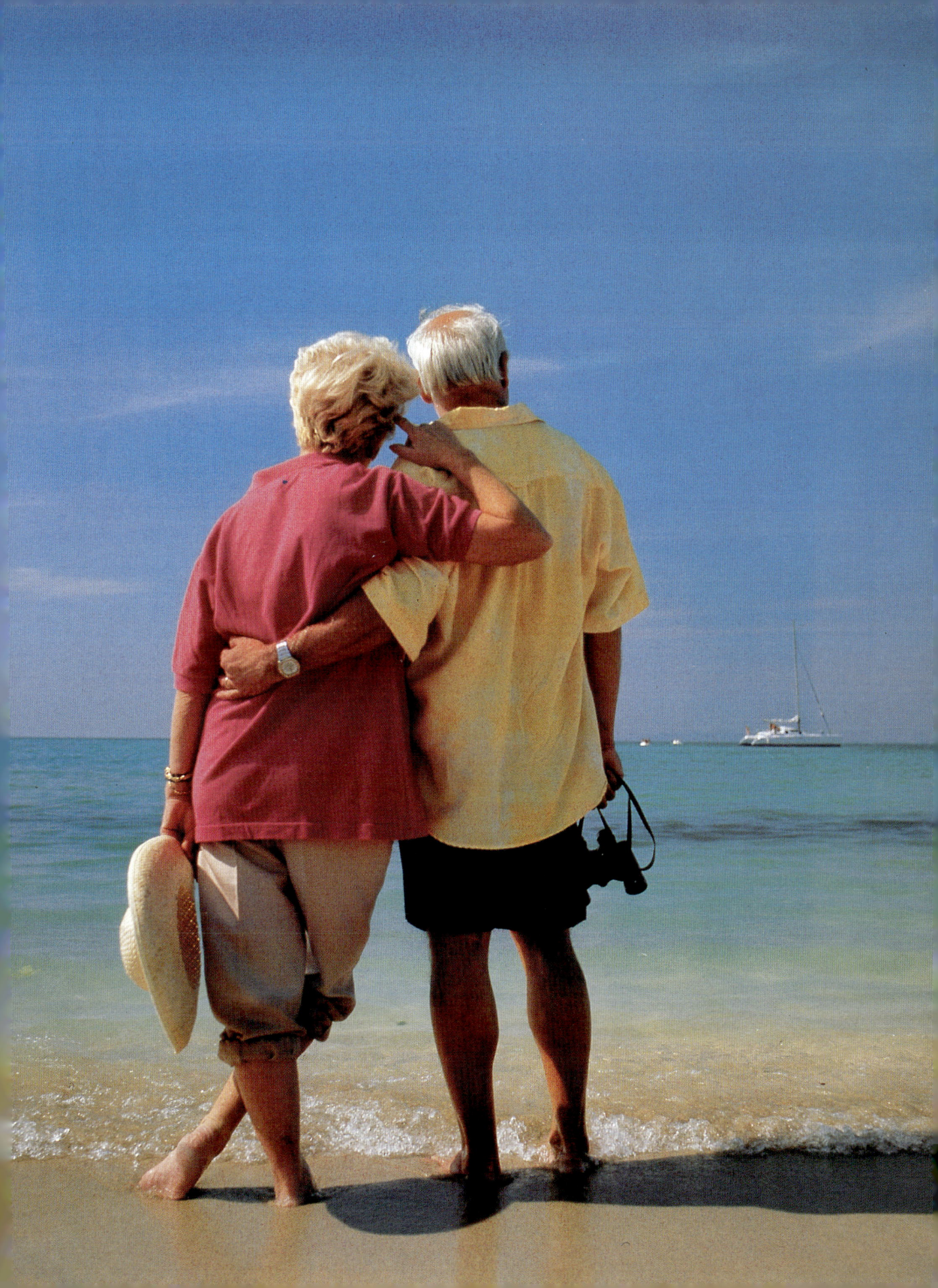

Sex Techniques & Practices

On the face of it, you might think that sex techniques would be the same the world over. There can't be that many different ways for people to get it together... can there? Think again! There are over 800 different cultural groups on this globe, and many of them have come up with an aspect of sex and loving that could give you some new ideas and quite a few new experiences.

Delving into some of the varied sex techniques enjoyed around the world may whet your appetite and put some sparkle into your sex-life

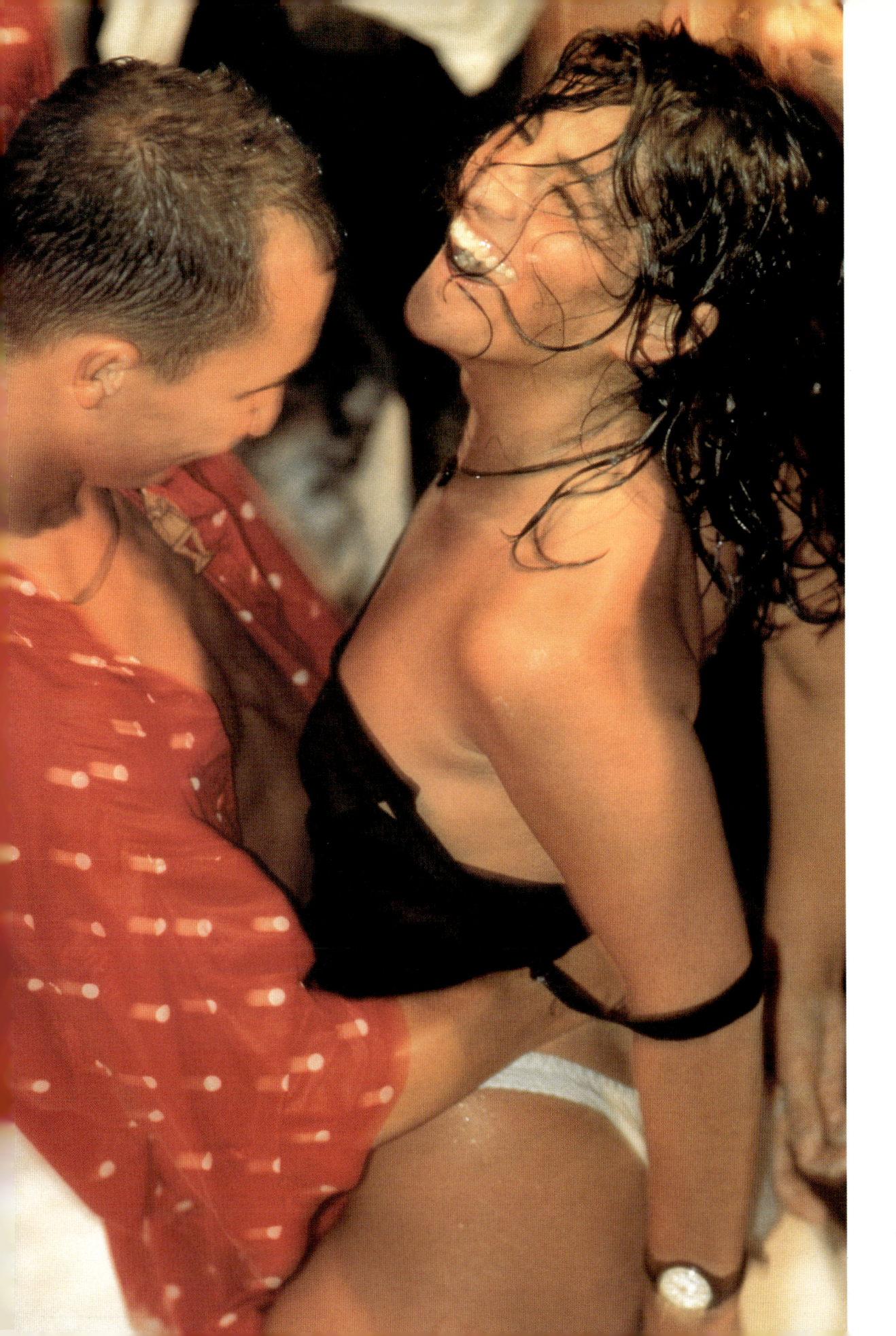

The modern West seems to be a unique culture in the way it approaches sex. This is influenced by the fact that it is, in general, more repressive about sexual matters than many other countries. Hidden impulses may therefore break out in certain sexual interests – interests not found in other cultures. For example, sado-masochism mostly stays within northern Europe and the USA, as does fetishism – obsessions with things such as rubber, high-heeled shoes and leather. Other cultures have pillow books on the arts of love, the West has pornography.

OTHER PEOPLE DO THE NAUGHTY BITS

Some societies, such as the Ila of south-east Africa, the Tukano of South America and the Trukese of the Pacific, have no word for virgin. However, this is not because sexuality is rampant or necessarily starts early in these groups, but because virginity is seen as an unimportant, transient state. Most human societies see sex as a normal part of life and a life without sex as positively abnormal. Abstinence – holding back from having sex on certain days or for certain periods in your life – is common. But being celibate, that is, not having a partner and not having sex at all, is widely held to be dangerous, unhealthy, tragic and highly peculiar.

A question of taste

Your diet can affect the taste of your body fluids. The semen and vaginal fluid of people whose diet is high in meat will have a more bitter taste than that of people who are largely vegetarian.

SEXUAL POLITICS

The Chinese were once renowned for their serious and intense approach to the arts of love. Since the revolution, the communist regime

WHATEVER SEXUAL TECHNIQUES AND PRACTICES YOU CHOOSE TO EXPLORE, YOU SHOULD ALWAYS TRY TO DISCUSS THINGS OPENLY WITH YOUR PARTNER TO MAKE SURE THAT YOU ARE BOTH COMPLETELY HAPPY AND RELAXED ABOUT WHAT YOU ARE DOING

cultivates an ethic that insists that sex wastes time and energy and diverts a citizen's commitment to the state. In Russia, things have changed rapidly since the break-up of the Soviet Union, although it is still one of the most sexually repressed societies in the world. Before the break-up, sex education was frowned on, pornography was banned and sex was seen as something that needed to be brought under control. Today, pundits prepared to speak about sex and offer advice are springing up on television and on the radio, and orgasm workshops have become popular.

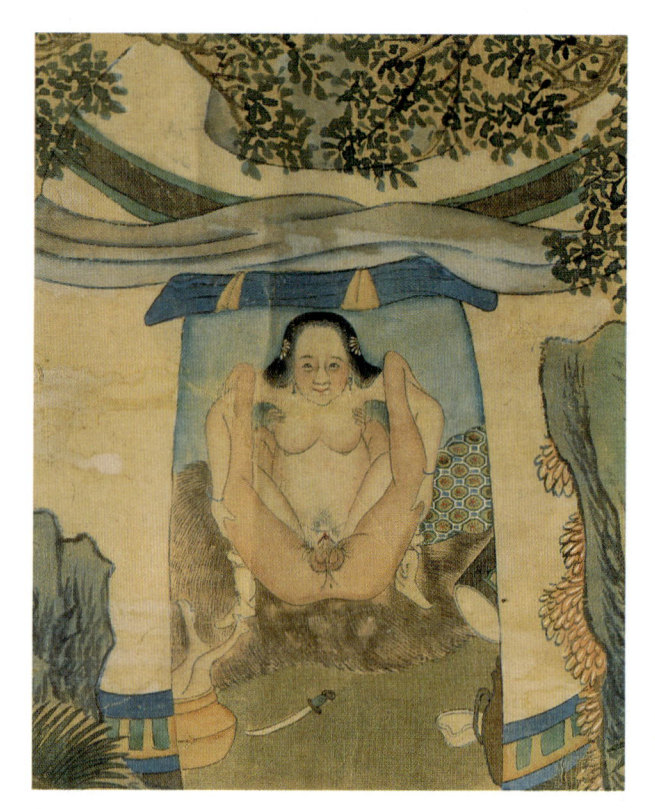

SKILLS IN LOVE WERE ONCE A CHINESE ART FORM, AND CHINESE "PILLOW BOOKS" OFTEN GRAPHICALLY DEPICTED ALL KINDS OF SEXUAL POSITIONS

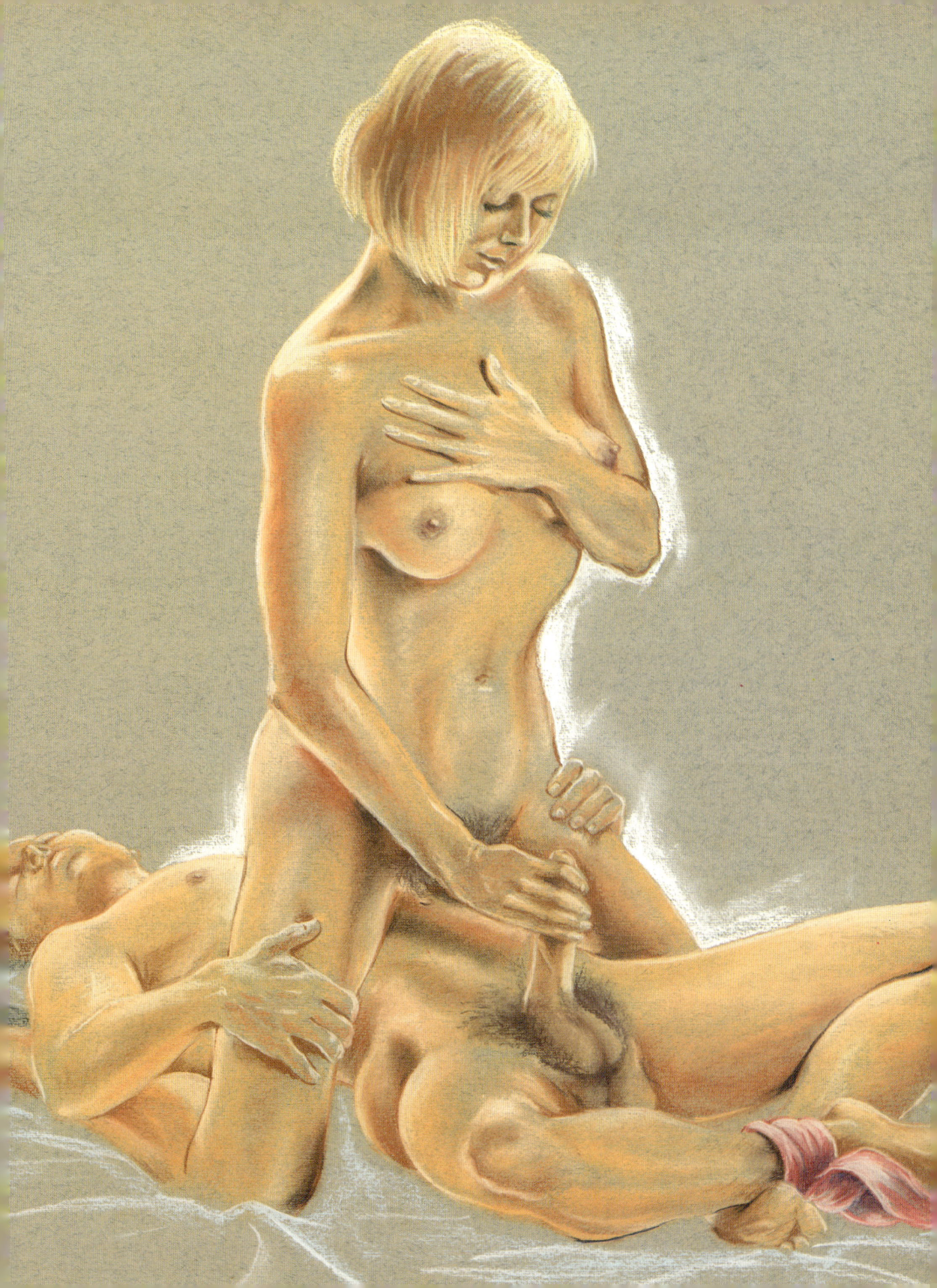

What's the secret?

A European survey found that the Danes think the secret of a good relationship is sharing the housework; the Spanish think it's children; the Irish believe a good wage makes all the difference; and the French swear by the distance you put between you and your in-laws. The Germans thought that sex was the least important aspect of marital harmony and only the British put it at the top of the list.

SACRED AND PROFANE

In the Balkans, rural men divide women into two categories – sacred and profane. Your mother, your wife and your sister are sacred. Profane women include gypsies, prostitutes, café singers and foreigners – especially Scandinavian tourists. Sex with your wife may be pleasurable, but it's certainly not regarded as fun because wives can't act or be treated the same way as a profane woman. Fun is to be had only with "bad girls".

People in the West may be tempted to think that this attitude means that societies everywhere else in the world are at it all the time! The truth is that, far from having a more promiscuous time of it, many cultures have very strict rules about when couples can have sex. These may result in men and women having to abstain from sex for more than half their reproductive life. In rural Bangladesh, for instance, 80 days a year are no-sex days because of rituals or festivals. In Hindu societies, you shouldn't have sex during certain phases of the moon. Among the Ivaro Native Americans, it's forbidden after planting narcotic plants, and among traditional Chinese there should be no sex on the birthdays of the gods. In various parts of Africa, sex during a thunderstorm, just before a fishing expedition or during daylight hours is a no-no.

Every society has sexual taboos. That is, an act, a word or an action that is just not done in polite society. In some societies, such as in the West, the penalty for breaking a taboo may be to be ostracized or to be tut-tutted and ignored by those around you. In others, breaking a taboo may actually be punished by death. What is taboo in one society can be perfectly normal in another. For instance, among the Yucatec and Mayan South Americans, you shouldn't have sex out of doors, and in Papua New Guinea, you shouldn't have sex indoors. And in the West, using certain gestures, such as "the finger", having sex with animals and anal sex is not at all the done thing.

Sex with animals is considered to be wrong in quite a few societies, and in some is punishable with a jail sentence. But among the Kuguru in Africa, it's just bad manners and inappropriate use of personal property. Muslims have a rule against all sex with animals but in Turkey some people regard it as sinful only when it involves animals that can be eaten, such as cattle or sheep. Turkish and Rif boys believe that sex with a donkey will increase the size of the penis – theirs, that is.

KISSY KISSY

To illustrate the great differences between many cultures around the world, let's look at kissing. You might think a peck on the cheek or a serious bout of tongue stroking is a pretty widespread way of showing affection. Wrong!

Kissing may be almost universal in the Western, Arab and Hindu societies, but it's totally unknown among the Somali, Cewa, Lepcha, Siriono and Sambia in Africa. The Inuit in the north, Tamils from Sri Lanka, the Ulithi, the Andamenese, Trobriand Islanders, the Thai, the Vietnamese and the Maoris rub noses, not only as a form of greeting, but also when they want to show sexual affection. The Thonga of Mozambique think kissing is an absolutely revolting habit because it means one person comes into contact with another's saliva. In Borneo, people sniff each other and the Ainu in Japan don't kiss but bite as their sign of affection. And, instead of kissing, groups such as the Tallensi of Ghana show affection by giving gifts.

Public propriety

In Kuwait, it is a criminal offence to kiss in public. Serbian women in Montenegro must defer to men at all times and husbands and wives are forbidden to show any form of affection when they are out.

In other countries, kissing and caressing on the mouth and with the mouth are considered to be one of the most delightful and sensual acts possible. If you have ever wondered why deep mouth kissing is called "French kissing", it's probably because of the Maraichins. They are from Brittany in France and they invented *Maraichinage*, the form of kissing in which lovers' tongues caress the insides of each other's mouths for long periods. *Maraichinage* can go on for hours. Do it right, and it may lead to an orgasm. The average kiss can burn up twelve calories. Done correctly, French kissing may mean you never have to diet again.

According to Tantric and Taoist beliefs, found throughout Asia and the Far East, the upper lip is one of the most sexy areas in the body. In fact, Hindu sex books claim that in women there is a nerve that runs directly from the upper lip to the clitoris. It's hardly surprising, therefore, that kissing is recommended as a way of arousing a woman's sexual urges and of driving her into a frenzy, prepared for love.

Tongue sushi

Why not try some serious kissing? Settle down with your partner, somewhere comfortable where you know you won't be disturbed. Make an agreement that kissing is all you are going to do – no touching, no intercourse. Now, see how far you can drive each other wild just by using your lips.

- *Try little, feathery-light kisses. Do them at the side of the mouth; do them dead centre.*
- *Try licking and sucking your partner's lips.*
- *Very gently, nibble and nip your partner's lips and around their mouth.*
- *With your tongue, gently stroke inside your partner's mouth; just inside their lips and deeper too, around the inside of their cheeks and their tongue.*
- *Gently and then more strongly, thrust your tongue inside their mouth, imitating the sexual thrusts of lovemaking.*

When you have recovered from all that, tell your partner which bits you really liked and which didn't do much for you, and listen to what they choose as favourites. Then, try it again!

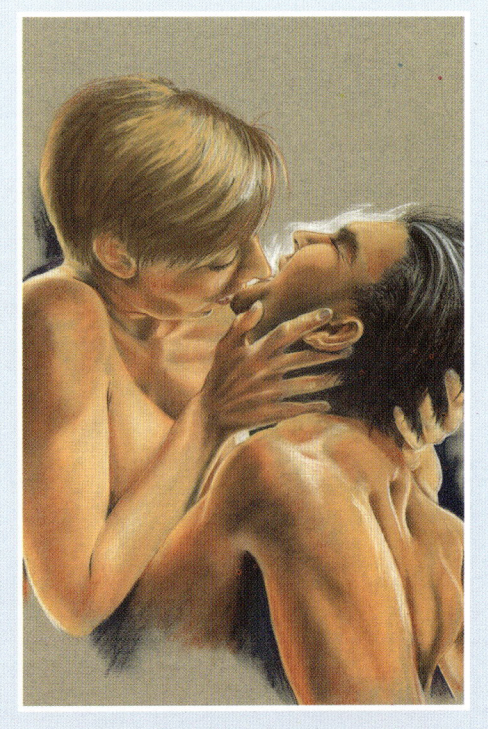

DRIVE EACH OTHER WILD WITH YOUR LIPS

CHASTE OR CHASED?

In some societies, sex is seen as a powerful and rather destructive force that must be kept under control. Others view it as a positive, life-enhancing influence. The Tanzanian Gogo believe that sex calms body and soul and that denying yourself the pleasures of love is positively unhealthy. In many societies, the main aim of marriage is to produce children and infertility is a reason for divorce, but Gogo men are just as likely to keep a wife they loved and who gave them sexual pleasure even if she was barren. Like them, the Makonde, also from Tanzania, expect both sexes to be expert at lovemaking. Makonde girls learn about sex through stories and talks from the elder women and are taught how to perform seductive dances for their menfolk.

The Zanzibaris expect a woman to be a virgin when she gets married and young girls are kept in seclusion in case sexual curiosity gets the better of them. Both sexes are taught how to please each other in bed and are expected to be faithful when they marry – fidelity for the men meaning to his group of wives, since the Zanzibaris are traditionally polygamous.

Among the Sarakatsani shepherds of Greece, women are not expected to enjoy sex at all but to lie back and be quiet. In fact, a bride is often expected to threaten her husband with dire injury when he comes to claim her virginity to show how inexperienced she is. The Sarakatsani also think male virginity is magical and special. A soldier who is still a virgin is considered to be invulnerable even to bullets.

FIRST-TIME SEX

Most of us remember the first time we had sex. It may have been romantic, wonderful and exciting. It may have been embarrassing, painful and disastrous. In some cultures, young people are prepared for their first experience by hearing dirty jokes, vague warnings and dire predictions about what it will be like. In others, they may be taught and allowed to practise in order to enjoy the event.

The mystical teachings of the East say that the first experience of sex is an important time, with more significance often for the girl than the boy. It's seen as a religious rite, so boys are initiated into the arts of love by experienced older women and are then urged to pass their knowledge and care on to a woman when she has her first experience with them. The man is taught to see himself as a representative of the Lord Shiva, god of regeneration, and to treat the woman like a goddess.

VARIETY IS THE SPICE OF SEX, AND BEDS ARE NOT THE ONLY FURNITURE YOU CAN USE TO TRY OUT A VARIETY OF POSITIONS AND ADD INTEREST TO YOUR LOVEMAKING

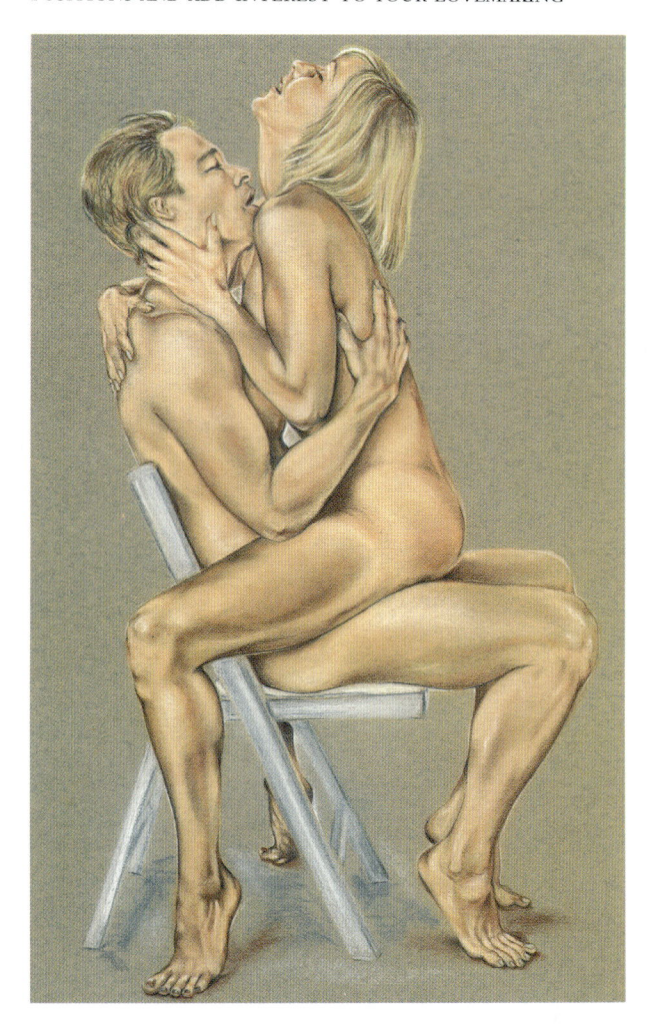

Love rite

The Kama Sutra describes a Tantric love rite which, if followed properly, guarantees sexual satisfaction for both partners:

1) Prepare your surroundings. Make sure that where you are going to make love is pleasant, comfortable and warm. Perfume the air with flowers, incense or scent. Dim the lights, have candles burning and put a dreamy tape or CD on. Have sexy nibbles – fruit, wine and some luxury treats – on hand.

2) Bathe or shower together. Have warm towels ready and rub each other dry. Spread the towels on your bed, the bathroom floor, the kitchen table or wherever takes your fancy. Now, lie down with your partner, take a generous handful of oil or cream and massage it all over your partner's body.

3) Take it in turns to kiss and stroke your partner's entire body SLOWLY from toes to head and back down again.

4) Make your caresses sexual. Concentrate now on your partner's favourite bits – and if you aren't sure which those are, ask!

5) Only when you have covered your partner's whole body with gentle caresses and luscious kisses can you go on to intercourse. Slowly and gently begin penetration, using a variety of sexual positions until both of you have experienced a climax. See the next chapter for ideas on sexual positions you can try!

HELP EACH OTHER TO REALLY ENJOY LOVEMAKING BY SLOWLY STROKING YOUR PARTNER'S FAVOURITE BITS

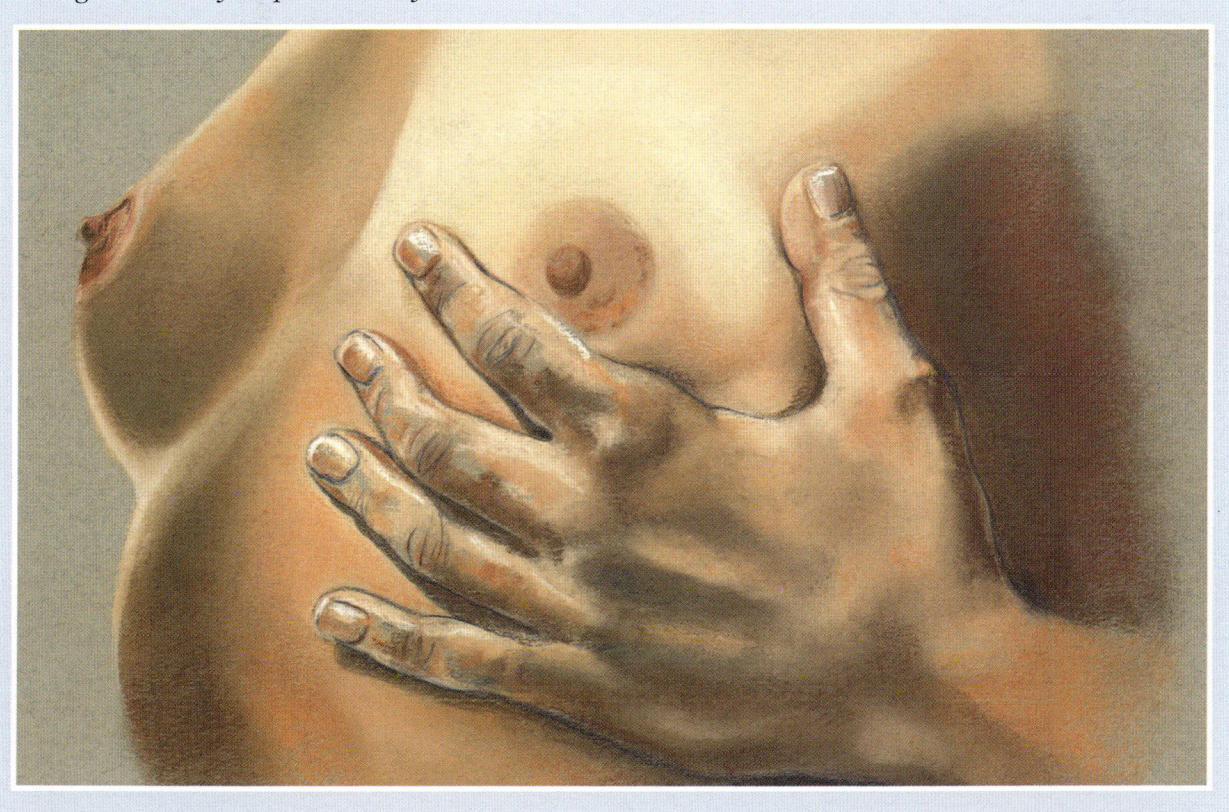

TANTRA AND TAO

Learning about Eastern sexual teachings and practices could do wonders for sex in the West. Some groups, particularly Hindus and Buddhists, believe that sexual intercourse is a spiritual act that allows a mystical union with a god. However, while sex is celebrated, losing semen is frowned on because it is believed to be the source of bodily strength. Both Tao and Tantric beliefs state that semen contains a man's energy and that expending it reduces his strength and may even shorten his life. Taoist masters recommend that a man should only ejaculate two or three times in every ten times he makes love. To this end, they recommend various techniques to help him make love for extended sessions and climax many times without ejaculating – it's ejaculation, not orgasm, that makes a man's penis deflate. These techniques are called *Karezza* and involve breath control, meditation and finger pressure on the penis to pull him back from the brink of ejaculation. Certain postures are recommended, such as sitting, squatting or lying on his back, as giving greater control over lovemaking and to direct energy to the brain. When he is really experienced, he is supposed to only ejaculate one in a hundred times.

But if Tantric and Taoist masters believe that losing semen is weakening, they also insist that absorbing female secretions goes a long way towards counteracting this weakening effect. So, making love for hours is supposed to be particularly good for men, because even though it may physically tire him and lead him to spend semen, at the same time he'll be taking in his partner's "yin" essence. She, in her turn, absorbs and is strengthened by his "yang" essence. So, next time anyone tells you you're sex mad, just point out that you're simply doing it for your health's sake!

IT IS ONLY BY EXPERIMENTATION THAT YOU WILL COME TO LEARN FULLY ABOUT YOUR OWN – AND YOUR PARTNER'S – BODY. SO, START FINDING OUT WHAT TURNS YOU BOTH ON!

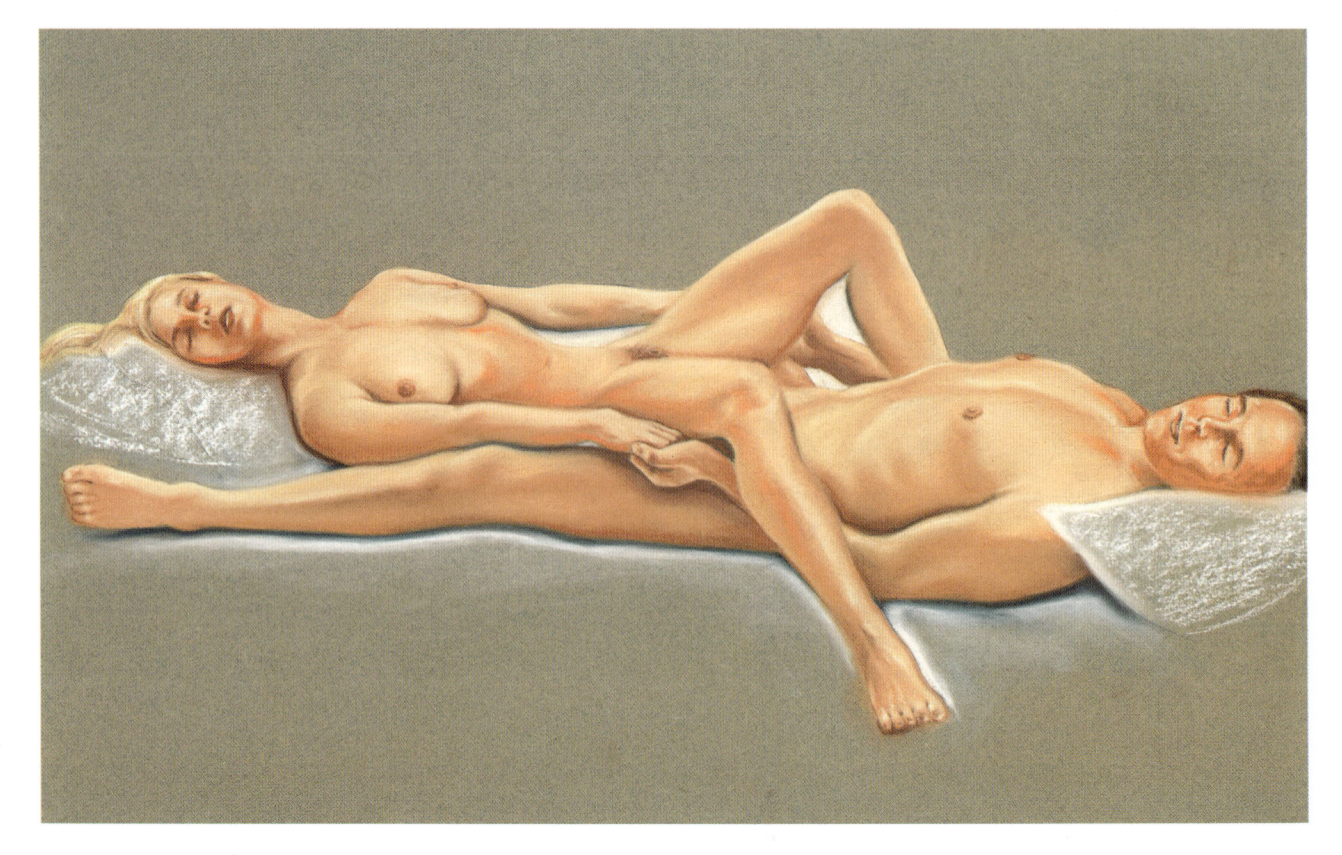

Gichigich technique

The Yapese, from Oceania, have a sexual technique called gichigich. *The woman sits in the man's lap and he puts his erect penis between her legs. He doesn't enter her vagina but slowly rubs himself between her labia and around the clitoris. Needless to say, this is extremely arousing and satisfying for her and women may reach multiple climaxes before the men finally come, too. Among the Yapese,* gichigich *is usually only used before marriage. Men say this is because it is so very exhausting. Once the couple are married and the woman less worried about pregnancy, they are likely to have ordinary, "missionary position" sex.*

TO SLEEP, TO DREAM

In the USA, gurus teach "sexual dreaming", promising a way of exploring your deepest desires. In fact, this suggestion is well-founded. Research shows that 80% of men and 40% of women have orgasms while they are asleep. All the fears and inhibitions that hold you back from fully enjoying yourself are absent at this time. In addition, many people have experienced the phenomenon of directive dreaming, when you can dictate what happens in a dream. It is easy to see how you can use this technique to enliven your dreaming sex-life! Research suggests that dreaming occurs during REM (rapid eye movement) periods of your night's sleep. On average you will have four or five sessions a night - enough time to enjoy your wildest fantasies.

Schools for sex

Do we need help in learning how to come? In Russia, they are holding orgasm workshops to help people who have never learned to enjoy sex to unlock their sensual potential. "Working Out" has a whole new meaning with American experts urging us to flex those "sex muscles", promising that multiple orgasms are possible for men and women if you do.

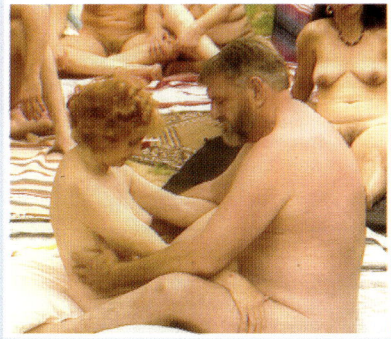

IN TANTRIC SEX WORKSHOPS, COUPLES CAN SHARE FANTASIES AND EXERCISES SO THAT THEY REAWAKEN THEIR SEXUAL SENSES

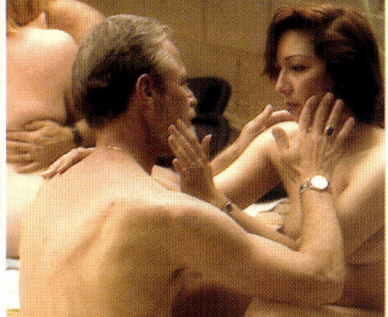

ENTHUSIASTS SAY THAT TOUCHING AND CARESSING SOMEONE YOU HAVE ONLY JUST MET RELEASES YOU FROM YOUR ANXIETIES AND INHIBITIONS

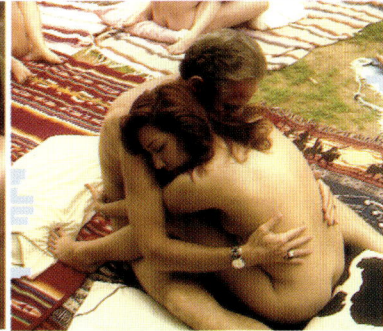

THE CLOSENESS THAT THESE WORKSHOPS ALLOW YOU TO BUILD UP WITH OTHER PARTICIPANTS CAN BE COMFORTING AS WELL AS SEXY

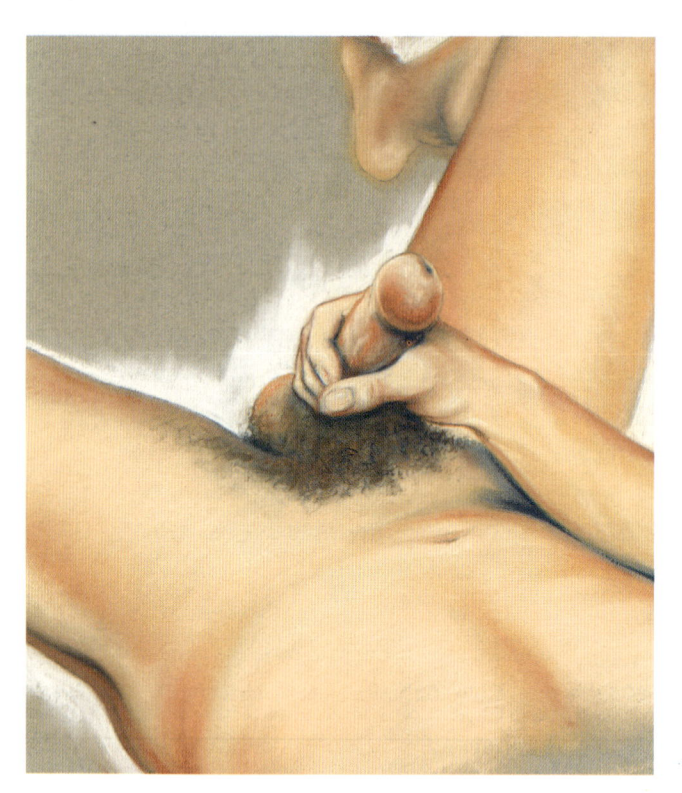

IT'S FUN, IT'S EXCITING, AND IT'S SEX WITH THE PERSON WHO KNOWS YOU BEST! MANY PEOPLE ENJOY MASTURBATION EVEN WHEN IN A LOVING AND SATISFYING SEXUAL RELATIONSHIP

SOLO SEX

Some cultures see self-pleasing or masturbation as a natural and normal part of sexual expression. It may be seen as the first and obvious way we explore our bodies and learn how they respond to touch. It can also be accepted as a common way of enjoying ourselves, either when we have no sexual partner with us, or when we want something different from shared caresses. Sadly, some other cultures see masturbation as wasteful or perverted. This is particularly true of religions which insist that sex is for creating new life and condemn any sexual activity that doesn't give rise to the possibility of pregnancy. Studies suggest that most men and women in Europe and the USA have masturbated and that it is a common form of sexual pleasure, not only for young people but also for older, married and partnered men and women.

A LITTLE SELF-SATISFACTION

Masturbation is sex with the person who knows you best. It can be a deeply comforting or exciting experience and one that can satisfy you at the time, or teach you for the future. You should never be ashamed or guilty about pleasing yourself. Many people in normal, happy relationships masturbate by themselves on occasions. It doesn't have to mean they love their partner any less or that they are missing anything in their shared love life. Sex can be like food in this respect – sometimes you want to grab a quick snack; sometimes you want to linger over a feast; sometimes you want to share a meal and sometimes you want to treat yourself, by yourself.

Treat yourself

Treat yourself to a bit of solo loving, and find out why the Kajaba recommend it so much! Make sure you have some private time. Run a bath and lock the bathroom door, or make sure everyone is out and you have the bed or sofa to yourself. Take your time, don't hurry. Lather your hands with soap or splosh a handful of cream or oil and slowly spread it all over your body. Stroke, rub and knead your whole body, from your head to your toes. Now, explore and stroke around your genitals, discovering and concentrating on whichever areas feel especially nice. Use gentle scratches, squeezes, palm and finger strokes; light, firm and hard caresses. As you come near to orgasm, concentrate on what you need to tip you over. Relax, and enjoy it. Remember what you did that was particularly pleasant and if or when you next make love with a partner, show them.

FACE THE MUSIC

Music and sex is a potent combination. Plenty of societies use dancing as part of religious ceremonies, but it is often a prelude to another form of rhythmic movement. The terms we use to describe music or dancing are frequently sexual. "Rock and roll", for instance, actually means "sexual intercourse" among the American black community who invented it! Among the Aranda, a native Australian group, the women dance when there are visitors, not only to entice the men but also to get their own juices flowing. When everyone is hot and sweaty, the women will get their husbands to fix a rendezvous with the men of their choice.

Why does music and dancing get us going? It does seem one of the few forms of sexual display that is common throughout the world. There is really very little difference between a tribal dance in the African bush and a local hop in an American town. Both do the same thing – allow groups of men and women to eye each other up and attract the attention of the people they fancy. They all have the same effect – to raise the temperature and turn minds to thoughts of love. And they frequently end up in the same way – with couples off in the bushes doing their own private version of the boogie.

One explanation is that music duplicates the pounding rhythm of the heart. You usually only hear your own pulse. Making love is the only time, as an adult, that you may be intimately aware of someone else's heartbeat. So, the thump of feet or a drum is an unconscious reminder of sex, putting you in the mood without your really realizing it. When you become sexually excited, your heartbeat speeds up, your temperature increases, you sweat, flush and pant. Dancing has the same effect, so putting the two together in your mind is obvious! When two people dance close together, with their bodies heating up and sweat trickling, it's really just a foretaste of pleasures to come.

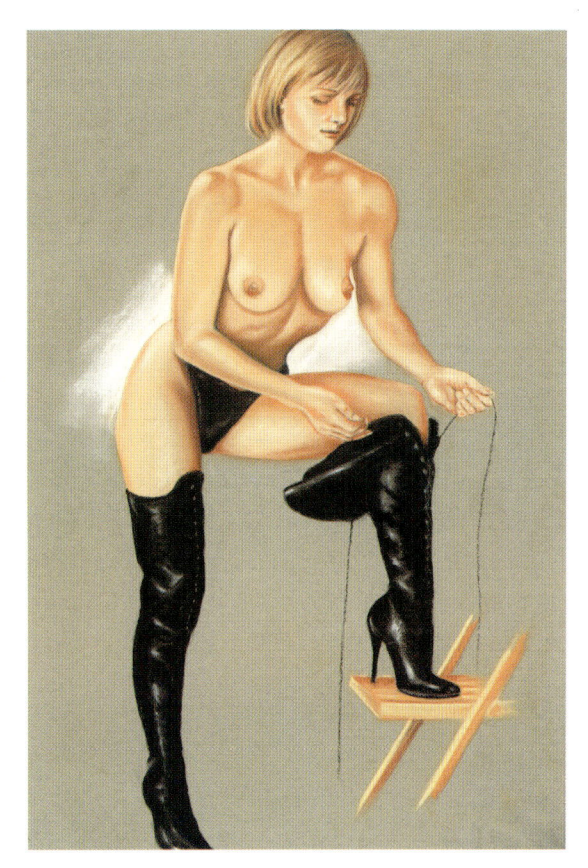

A TOUCH OF FETISHISM CAN LIVEN THINGS UP

ROUGHING IT

Just as dancing raises the pulse and temperature and prepares the way for sex, so too does a scare or a row. This is partly why horror and violence have become so popular in many aspects of the Western media. When you get frightened, the adrenalin starts flowing and you also become sexually aroused. Fast driving is a sexual thrill, and so is fighting. Sometimes these risk behaviours are a form of foreplay, sometimes they're a substitute for the real thing. Joining the "Mile High Club" by making love in a plane may be an exclusively Western way of scaring the pants off each other, as is going to the theme park and spending the afternoon on a rollercoaster, but other cultures raise the pulse with equally effective means.

S and M (sado-masochism), with its leather and rubber clothing, straps, chains and buckles, is something that the northern and eastern

SEX TECHNIQUES & PRACTICES

Europeans seem to do so well and like so much. Punishment, particularly beatings, have always been a part of the Western, Christian tradition's emphasis on doing penance.

You don't have to go as far as the dedicated SM enthusiast to like a bit of rough love. Some people find that treating the body roughly can be fun. And so it can be if it's to your taste and is done with proper care and safety. What is central to rough sex is that you and your partner both really choose to do this, and that you both keep an element of control. There is nothing sexy or exciting about one person using force or coercion against another to get their thrills. When real violence and fear are present, it isn't sex and it isn't love – it's simply a crime and an abuse. But many people do find that pain and pleasure can be surprisingly close, and that the illusion of dominating or being dominated adds sexual excitement.

Try it

A common form of light SM is bondage. Why don't you and your partner try the simplest form of bondage tonight? Use a tie, belt or scarf to bind one of you to the bed, or to the sofa. Then play-act being dominated by or dominating your partner.

If you want to extend your SM fantasies, you can improvise or buy all kinds of equipment and clothing. There are blindfolds and gags, chains and padlocks, and leather wrist and ankle cuffs and collars. You can have ropes, straps, chains and custom-made harnesses that tie hands behind the back or to the waist, thighs, ankles or neck, or can be used to tie your partner to the bed, floor or ceiling. (Check that the structure won't come apart in a passion-killing shower of plaster or splintering wood.)

Protecting your virtue

S and M enthusiasts can also buy – for both sexes – complete harnesses that are "chastity" barriers, that is, they prevent the wearer from being able to have sex. Genuine chastity belts are actually quite rare around the world. In the Caucasus, they wear a type of chastity corset, and the Yakut of north-eastern Siberia require their girls to wear leather trousers, tied on with multiple straps. These are supposed to be worn all the time, until she is married.

If you want to see whether rough sex turns you on, talk beforehand about how far you wish to go and what you want to do. Agree a word or phrase that you can use to stop the action immediately and without argument. Of course, the main excitement for some bondage enthusiasts lies in the very fact that they are unable to stop. One extreme example of this is the suggestion made by some enthusiasts that you send off the key in a stamped addressed envelope before snapping the padlock that fastens them into their bonds. While having the utmost respect for the postal service, this author thinks anyone who trusts it to this extent is crazy. If you are trying out this form of sexual adventure, have an escape route ready.

The grown-up baby

Another sexual interest that seems to arise mainly in northern Europe is the "grown-up baby" game. Played to the full, it involves adult men dressing in giant nappies, lying in cots and being fed, from bottle or breast, by their "mother". You may have seen advertisements for "nurseries" catering for this interest.

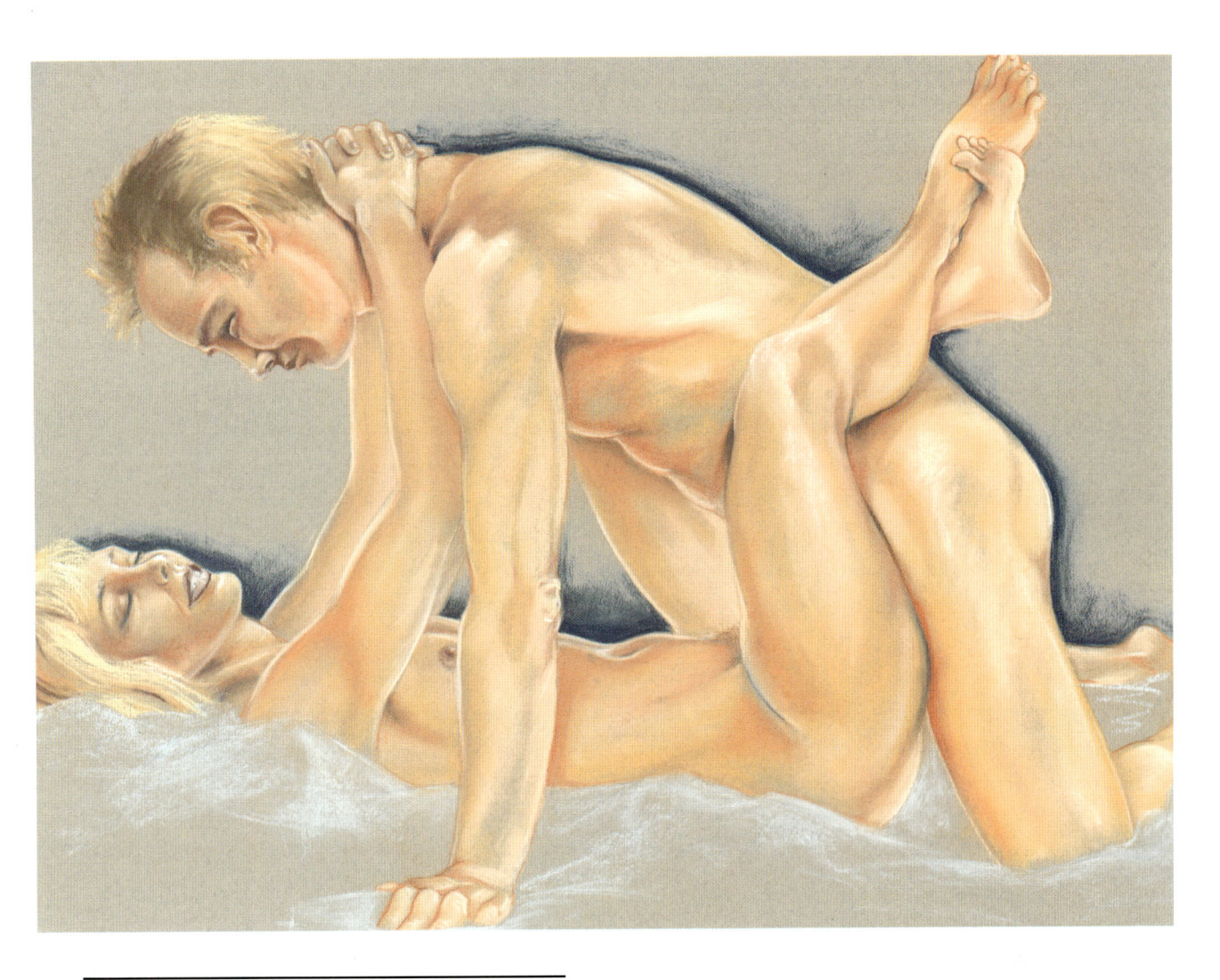

TIME AND TIME AGAIN

Human beings may not, like animals, have a season for mating, but it would seem that the time of year has some effect on our sexual behaviour. In Britain, it's said that "In the spring, a young man's fancy lightly turns to thoughts of love." However, it seems to take them about three months to really get going, because Westerners in America and Europe tend to have a birth bulge around March and April. This suggests that it's the summer holidays that are often a cue for lovemaking. In contrast, among the Inuit, more babies are born in late summer and autumn than at any other time of the year. This is because Inuits have sex far more often during the long winter nights than they do during the long summer days.

THE WARMTH OF A SUMMER CLIMATE ENCOURAGES MANY OF US TO RELAX AND INDULGE IN MORE SEX, AND EXPERIMENT WITH DIFFERENT POSITIONS. WHY NOT FANTASIZE ABOUT HAVING SEX ON THE BEACH – OR TRY IT FOR REAL!

Whenever we do it, do different cultures make love more often than others? Alfred Kinsey, in his major study of sex in America, found that an average frequency of sex was four times a week among teenagers, three times among thirty-year-olds, two for the forties and one for sixty-year-olds. Overall, he suggested that American couples make love an average of two to three times a week. In other cultures, frequency of sex can range from once a week among the Keraki of New Guinea to ten times a night for the Chaga of Tanzania.

Not tonight, dear...

There are plenty of beliefs about the dangers of sexual activity and particularly of sex done at the wrong time, in the wrong place or in the wrong position. Rabbis used to say, for instance, that sex standing up would lead to convulsions; sex sitting down would lead to delirium; on the floor to unhealthy children; and, in any position other than straight man-on-top, to diarrhoea! Italian soccer coaches ban their teams from having sex before a match. The belief that you shouldn't have sex before any sort of sporting activity is quite common, but the most thorough scientific study on sex and its effects shows that orgasm has hardly any effect on stamina or muscular strength at all. In fact, if anything, because it relaxes the body and promotes restful sleep, it could be said to improve performance. This isn't to say that orgasm can't have its harmful little side-effects – Attila The Hun, Nelson Rockefeller and Pope Leo the Eighth all died while having sex.

Not this year, dear...

Having children can cast a distinct pall over a couple's sex life. This can begin from the very moment your bundle of joy is on the way. The Kikuyu and Masai people believe sexual intercourse during pregnancy causes a miscarriage, a belief shared by many cultures. The Kikuyu allow sex, as long as the man only penetrates five centimetres inside his partner.

Probably the greatest fear in pregnant sex is that intercourse will damage the baby – what doctors call "foetal embarrassment". In fact, adult embarrassment is your greatest enemy – the lingering fear that all that humping is somehow being spied upon or incestuously shared by a tiny, innocent babe who can be harmed by the experience. On the contrary, developing babies do not need total quiet and stillness for a successful pregnancy, and it is thought that parental satisfaction is transmitted to a baby. Lovemaking is more beneficial than a tense, unwilling abstinence, but the way you make love may have to be different during pregnancy. (For the actual mechanics of intercourse during pregnancy, see Chapter 4.)

Current Western medical thinking sees pregnant sex as safe and desirable in a healthy pregnancy that is free from any complications, and where the man and the woman are both happy with the pregnancy and their relationship. The arguments that persist against it – that it can cause infection, premature labour or miscarriage – would seem to have more to do with cultural attitudes towards women and sex than with scientific fact.

Pregnancy can even improve a woman's sexual satisfaction. Three fifths of women in a recent survey said that their sex lives were either unchanged or bettered during pregnancy. If we weren't meant to have sex during a pregnancy, it is strange that we have evolved to enjoy it so much at this time. The increase in breast size during pregnancy can do wonders for many women's sexual self-esteem. In the vagina, the mucous membranes thicken and secretion increases. This vaginal congestion can mean that orgasm or multiple orgasm becomes easier, even though they may be less intense than in the non-pregnant state.

Some men – and women too – unconsciously put women in pigeon holes. Childless women can be seductive and enjoy sex, but The Mother is sacred and above that. As soon as a pregnancy is established, a man with this attitude may find himself unable to "desecrate" his wife with a sexual advance. Similarly, a woman may find the idea of sex somehow wrong. It is highly significant that pregnancy, especially if it is the first, is one of the most common times for men to wander sexually. The Bemba, an African people, have one very good way of stopping men roaming. They believe that if a man is unfaithful while his wife is pregnant, the baby will be stillborn.

Some couples find sex during pregnancy especially arousing, both emotionally and physically

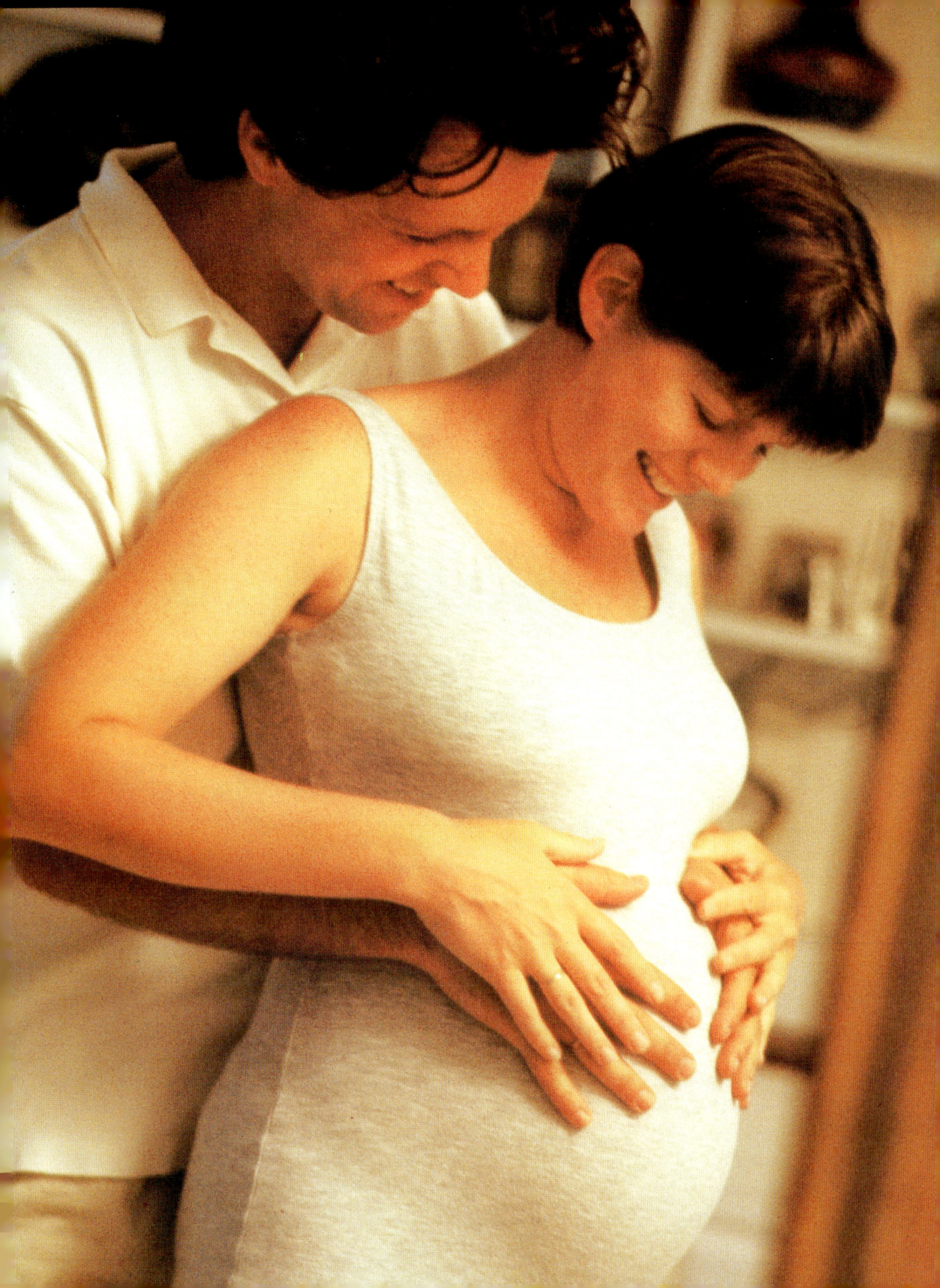

The time of your lives

Pregnancy can be one of the sexiest times in your life together. Many women find that the hormonal changes that take place produce a real sense of calmness and well-being, and this can combine with the sexual frisson caused by changes to the breasts and genitals to make her feel more voluptuous than ever before. She has proved her fertility and she is now also free of any of the constraints or inhibitions that went with birth control. The man, too, can share this mixture of pride and freedom, and many admit to a particular edge of sexual excitement in making love to a pregnant partner. This is probably added to by pheromones produced by the woman during pregnancy. These are the hormones that have a consciously or unconsciously detectable "sex smell". They are especially potent at this time and can increase sexual excitement in both the man and the woman.

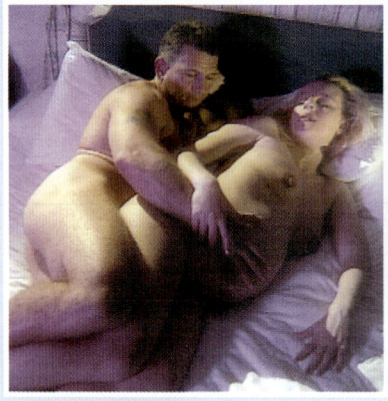

You will almost certainly have to use positions other than "man on top" during pregnancy, especially in the later stages

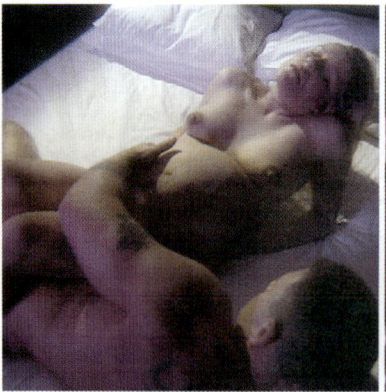

Pregnancy can increase a couple's sexual satisfaction, and slow, sensuous sex is good for mum, dad... and baby, too

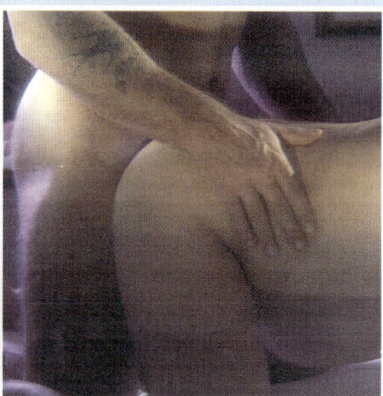

Rear entry and side-by-side positions give you a chance to get close and enjoy satisfaction in spite of that bulge

The food of life

In several South American cultures, sex in pregnancy is not only allowed, it's actually encouraged. Semen is thought to be nourishing for babies – indeed it's even believed to be the only food a developing baby gets. So loving, caring parents will make love as often as possible, right up until birth, to keep their baby from going hungry.

Most new parents do find that their sex life suffers under the strain of having children in the house. Only 29% of Western fathers with children (as opposed to 40% of men with no children, or whose children had left home) say they are happy with their sex life. Of men with a current sex problem, two out of five with children under five say it is directly connected to the pregnancy or the birth.

In Britain, women are generally advised to wait until the check-up six weeks after childbirth before considering having sex again. In the Yemen, women can resume their sex life forty days after a child is born. On that day the mother is bathed, perfumed and has designs painted on her hands and legs to celebrate her readiness. In reality, both women and their partners may not be in the mood by that time, although some may be raring to go. In other countries, the interval between childbirth and having sex again can be far greater. The Mende of Sierra Leone think semen and blood poison a woman's breast milk. She is not supposed to have sex until children are weaned. And in Sierra Leone, as in much of Africa, children are breastfed until they are two, three or even four years old. It's thought that the semen will penetrate the baby's feet and prevent them from walking. The practical side of such beliefs is that it enforces birth spacing. The down side is that husbands may pressure wives to hurry a child onto solid food so that they can get back to having sex.

The most obvious bar to marital bliss, especially in the first few years of being a parent, is that you are often too tired to think of doing anything more strenuous in bed than sleeping. Another common complaint, especially during the early days after childbirth, is that lovemaking is too painful. The muscles surrounding the vagina can not only be bruised during childbirth, but become strained and slack. These are the muscles that contract and spasm during sexual excitement and orgasm. The pelvic floor muscles are rather like a sling, stretching from the pubic bone to the coccyx (tail bone) and holding the pelvic organs in place. When the muscles are taut and firm, not only can you hold your urine when you want, but you can also hold your partner's penis in your vagina in a firm embrace.

As labour advances, the pregnancy hormone progesterone softens these muscles to allow them to stretch and let the fully grown baby pass through the cervix and down the vagina. If the muscles are not yet ready to allow this to happen, or if labour lasts for too long, the muscle tissue can get damaged and over-stretched, making it slack. When this happens, the woman may find that lovemaking loses some of its sensation, and she cannot feel her partner's penis inside her. He may complain of her vagina feeling loose and of his penis being "lost". Successive pregnancies, a traumatic birth and ageing can all serve to further the softening of these muscles. Although you cannot always avoid trauma, and you certainly can't avoid ageing, you can give yourself the best possible chance of retaining good muscle tone. Firm pelvic muscles in a firm and trim body are more likely to bounce back in fighting form after the passage of your baby. So, if you are to regain full pleasure in making love, it is worth getting these muscles into shape with exercises both before and after your pregnancy. (For information on sex muscle exercises, see Chapter 5.)

For ten to twelve weeks after giving birth, a woman is likely to find that her genitals will have undergone some temporary changes. She may find that vaginal lubrication is slower to flow during sexual excitement. In spite of feeling sexual desire, many women find that orgasm is far harder to reach, and could even elude them. It is almost as if the sexual tension has become slack, and takes longer to tune up. Breasts, however, can be even more sensitive than before, if the woman is breastfeeding. She may well find that sexual excitement triggers a flow of milk and that her breasts are far quicker to give her stimulation.

Breastfeeding is itself a highly sexual experience, a fact that confuses and even angers some women, and their partners. During suckling, the body responds to the pressure on the nipple by releasing a hormone called oxytocin. This stimulates milk flow, but it also has an effect on the uterus and the genitals. Some mothers find breastfeeding can bring them to orgasm, and that breast-play is highly exciting.

The change of status of his partner, from wife and lover to mother, can be a severe blow to the male libido, and some men even find their own bodies rebelling – they become impotent when faced with a sexual offer from the woman they now see as Mother and therefore taboo. Some can become so traumatized by the association of sex with the pain of childbirth, that their disgust or fear renders them incapable. Or, they may feel sexually willing but be too concerned for their partner's well-being to press their desires upon her. Pregnancy and birth are too often treated as if they were illnesses. If the couple don't talk honestly to each other about their desires, he may leave her alone out of a misplaced sympathy, while she feels too hurt to make a pass, thinking he has gone off her.

Getting back together

There are several measures you can take to make lovemaking pleasant between you again. Firstly, you should both recognize that, although you are now Mum and Dad, you are still partners, and lovers. In order to allow yourselves the opportunity to continue to feel this very special link, you need to make time and physical space to enjoy it. Babysitters – especially doting grandparents – should be used ruthlessly, not only to allow you to have the odd evening out together, but also the odd night in on your own, as well as weekends or holidays as a private couple.

Before intercourse becomes desirable or possible, both of you might find that non-penetrative sex brings back the language of love and touch to your life, and gives both of you a chance to cherish each other and relax. Rather than it being a sexual moratorium, the fact that you can't make full love could be a valuable learning experience, enabling you to find out how to bring mutual comfort and excitement in other ways.

LOVE, LOVE, LOVE

Attitudes vary across cultures to sex, love and marriage for very good reasons. Westerners may think those who are not bowled over by love are abnormal, or missing out on something. The opposite argument may be that romantic love is painful, obsessive and unrealistic. Far from being the norm, it is actually fairly unusual. Romantic love is a concept that is almost entirely confined to Europe and North America. One theory for its existence is that, in cultures where man and wife are tied by the dependence on each other for the basic necessities of life, romantic love is unnecessary. Where husband and wife have a degree of independence, a marriage may be more at risk. So, romantic love has grown up to keep them together. Luo and Yoruba women think sex is no big deal. Couples sleep in different rooms and may only have sex when a wife signals to her husband that it's the right time of the month for her to conceive a child. She does this by folding a banana leaf covering his food in a special way.

TAKE MY WIFE... PLEASE!

Quite a few societies practise sexual hospitality, when a visitor won't just be offered a good meal and a bed for the night as a welcome. He will also be offered the sexual use of his host's wife, or sometimes his daughter. This custom is found in Africa, Siberia, Alaska, Polynesia and the Aleutian Isles. Among the Koryak of north-east Asia, a man would be so insulted if a visitor turned down the offer of sex with his wife or daughter that he may kill the rude guest in retaliation.

Customs such as this may be fine for the men involved, but not such fun for the wives. Inuit women are subject to an hysterical state of

THE WESTERN IDEAL IS MUTUAL PLEASURE AND ROMANTIC LOVE, WHEREAS IN SOME OTHER CULTURES, SEX ONLY TAKES PLACE FOR MALE SATISFACTION OR TO PRODUCE CHILDREN

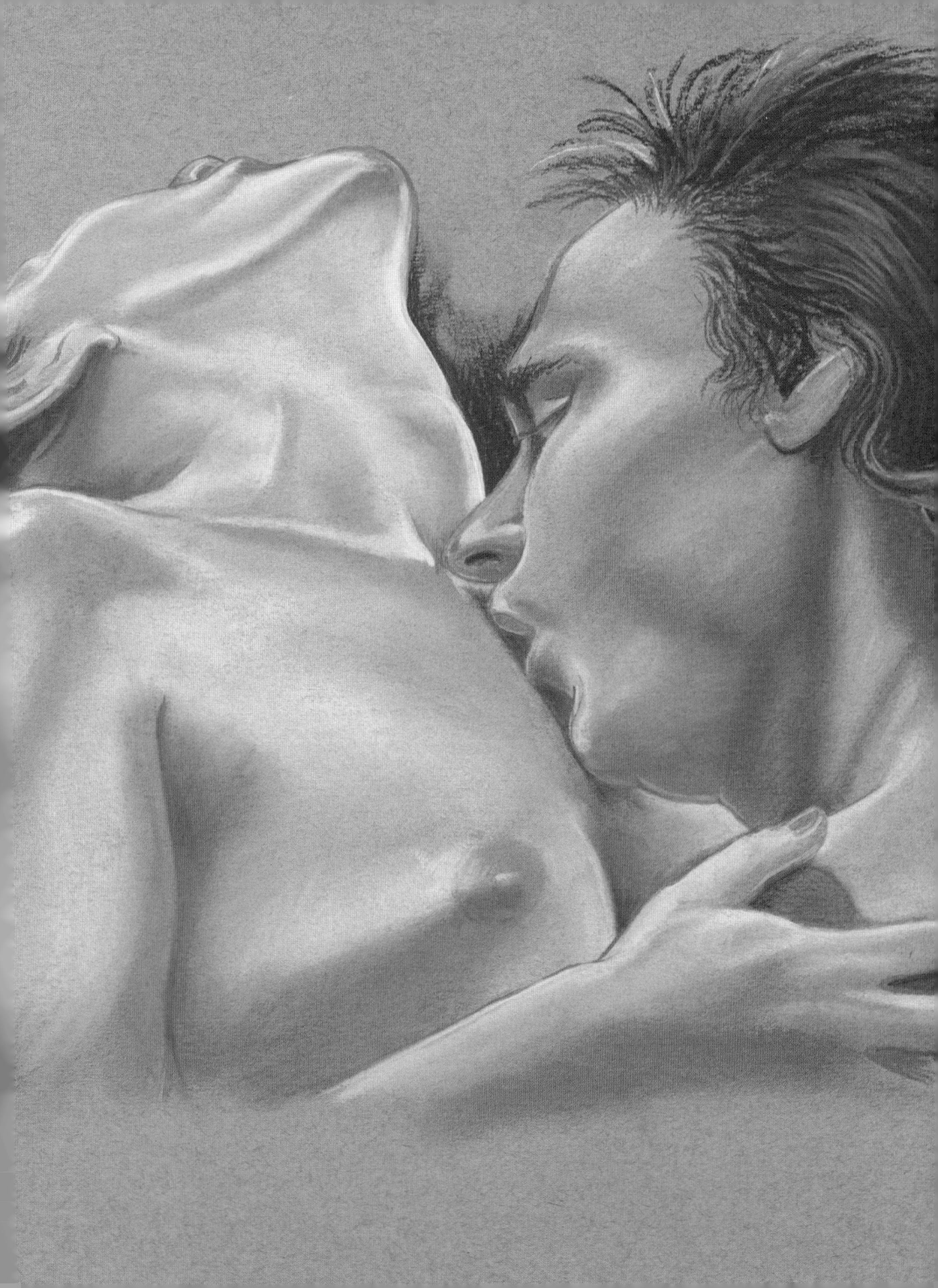

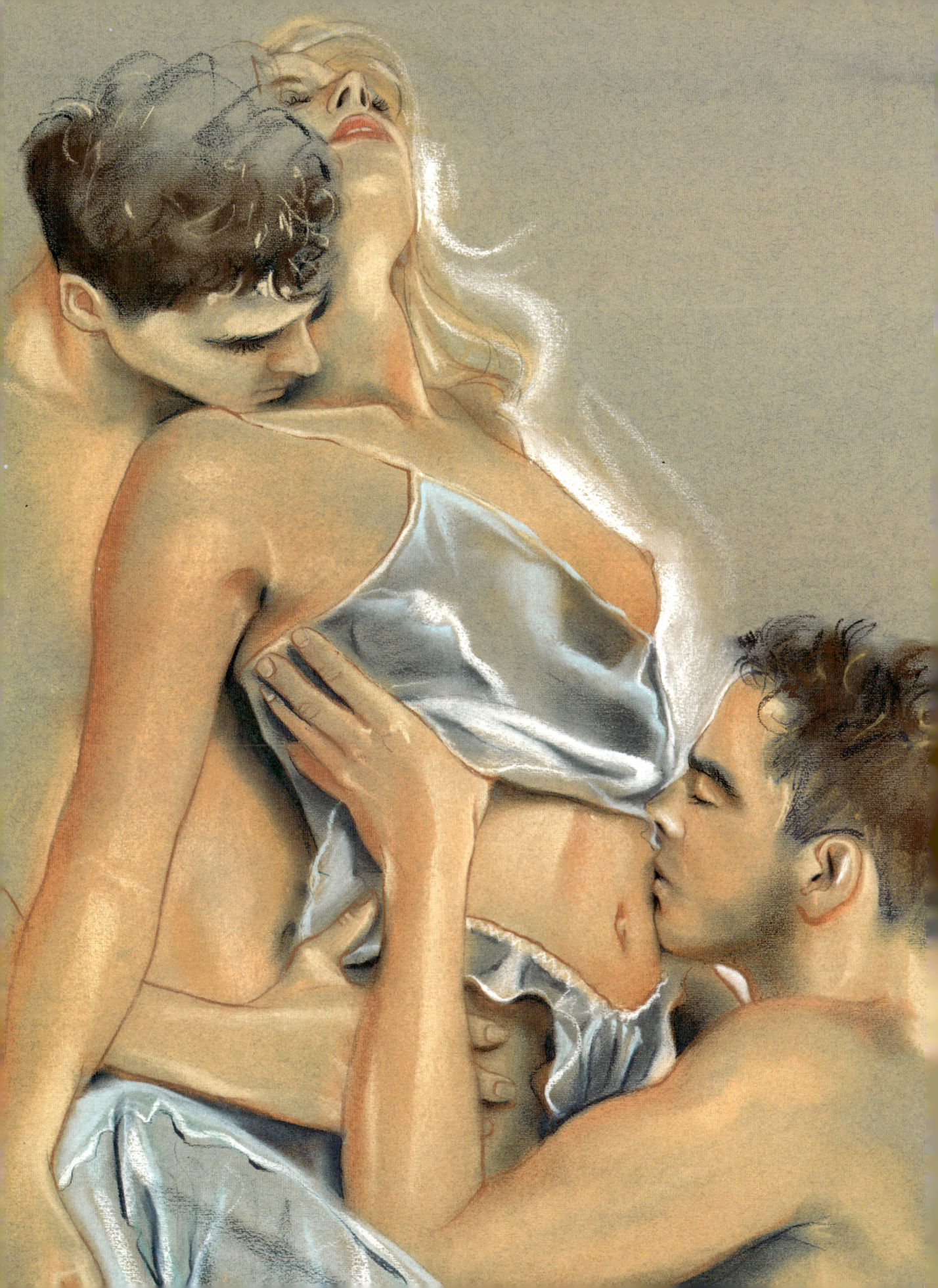

breakdown called *piblokto*, in which they tear off their clothing and run naked into the snow, screaming, before collapsing with total amnesia about what they've done. However, sexual hospitality isn't always at the invitation of husbands. A visiting Masai man may be invited to use one of his host's wives. Equally, a wife may herself extend the invitation and the sign that she has a visitor is his spear placed across the door of her dwelling. Her husband will respect her privacy and no questions are asked.

As has already been mentioned, one-to-one exclusive relationships are not the pattern of marriage and sexual relationships experienced by the majority of human cultures. Even in largely monogamous societies, people have affairs. After all, if you have a rule, there is always the temptation to break it.

It's often argued that an affair can have a beneficial emotional and sexual effect on the main relationship. Women can report having their first orgasm with a lover after years of unsatisfactory sex with partners, and that this often helps them to make married sex better. Some say that an affair gives them confidence and self-esteem and makes them feel sexually exciting and experienced. But in one study, while two out of three married men thought an affair would not be destructive to their marriage and that they would forgive or expect to be forgiven one, half of divorced men thought that fidelity was vital. When an affair does actually happen and is discovered, infidelity has the power to hurt more deeply than any other act between couples.

IN MANY NON-WESTERN SOCIETIES, MONOGAMY AND PRIVACY IN SEXUAL MATTERS WOULD BE CONSIDERED HIGHLY PECULIAR. TODAY, AN INCREASING NUMBER OF WESTERNERS ARE ALSO QUESTIONING THESE VALUES AND ARE TAKING PART IN VARIOUS TYPES OF GROUP SEXUAL ACTIVITY – ENTHUSIASTS SAY THAT THIS HAS GIVEN THEIR SEX-LIVES A MUCH-NEEDED BOOST

SWAPPING AND SWINGING

Swinging is when couples exchange partners. Partner-swapping happens all over the Western world. In effect, it's a way for people living in monogamous cultures to experiment with the sort of marital forms common in multi-partner societies. There are private clubs set up throughout Europe, Australia, New Zealand and the USA where couples can go to swing. Over a hundred clubs exist in Germany today offering group sex or partner swapping. In some cases, couples join a group and parties take place in each other's homes. Swinging can involve group sex. That is, couples might meet at swinging parties and have sex with whoever takes their fancy from those assembled. They can do this either in private in a separate room, or in public as part of the proceedings. Swinging may also involve two couples getting together for the purpose. Again, sex may then take place as a group or with each couple going off to separate rooms.

Swinging attempts to get round the emotional risks of extra-relationship sex, by making it a shared activity between the couple. Similarly, swinging parties keep the activity to a set time, so you experience sex without emotional commitment. And swapping between couples becomes a four-way involvement, rather than each partner going off to have their own separate sexual relationship outside.

However, if you have been brought up to see having one partner as the "right way", there are emotional risks to dabbling in other patterns. If one or other of the couple is going along to please or placate their partner, or if one enjoys the experience more than the other, jealousy and hurt can be the result. Don't forget that even when the accepted family arrangement is several wives to a husband or several husbands to a wife, participants say quarrels, jealousy and feelings of rejection are common. Where sex is not kept exclusively to a couple or between a married group, there are the physical risks, too. For an open marriage, or sexual activities involving other partners, to work, both members of a couple need to be responsible, careful and sensitive to each other's feelings and needs, as well as being concerned for and honest with their other sexual partners.

Sexual techniques are varied and various around the world, but one aspect of sex you might think can't have that many differences is how you actually get it together. After all, there are only so many ways you can have intercourse... aren't there? Wrong! There are literally hundreds of sexual positions you can attempt, and different cultures favour different ones. If you'd like to find out how they prefer to make love in Brisbane and Berlin, Archangel and Auckland, London and Louisville, then turn to the next chapter!

Safer swapping

If you want to involve other people in a couple relationship, take these simple but essential precautions:

1) Always use condoms and Safer Sex practices with any other partner.

2) Be honest and tell your partner if you are involved with someone else.

3) Stop any outside relationship if it takes up more time or emotional energy than your permanent one.

4) Stop any outside relationships if your partner has second thoughts.

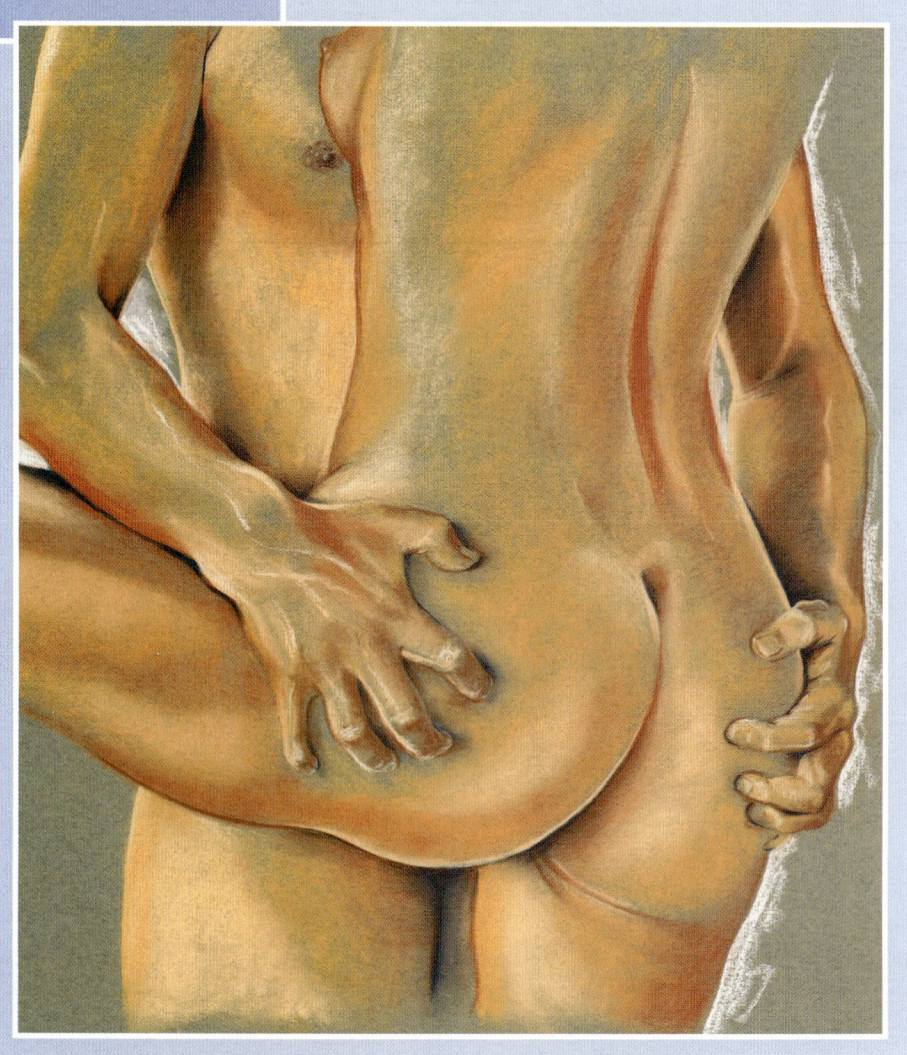

DON'T GET CARRIED AWAY BY THE EXCITEMENT OF PARTNER-CHANGING. SAFER SEX AND TOTAL HONESTY ARE VITAL PARTS OF SUCCESSFUL SWAPPING AND SWINGING

Putting on a condom

Use a new condom for each sexual encounter and put it on before any genital contact takes place. If the woman puts it on her partner, then it can become a part of making love, and doesn't interrupt the action or spoil any of the fun.

1) *Make sure that his penis is hard – you can't put a condom onto a soft penis.*

2) *Hold the condom by the closed end, squeezing the tip shut between thumb and finger to expel trapped air. Unroll the condom down the shaft of his penis.*

3) *Make sure that she's absolutely ready before you start making love. If she's not wet enough, the condom may tear. You might need the help of some suitable, water-based lubricant (such as KY jelly).*

4) *After he's come, hold the open end of the condom against the penis as he pulls out to make sure the condom doesn't slip off as he withdraws.*

5) *Tie a knot in the end of the condom, wrap it in a tissue and throw it away.*

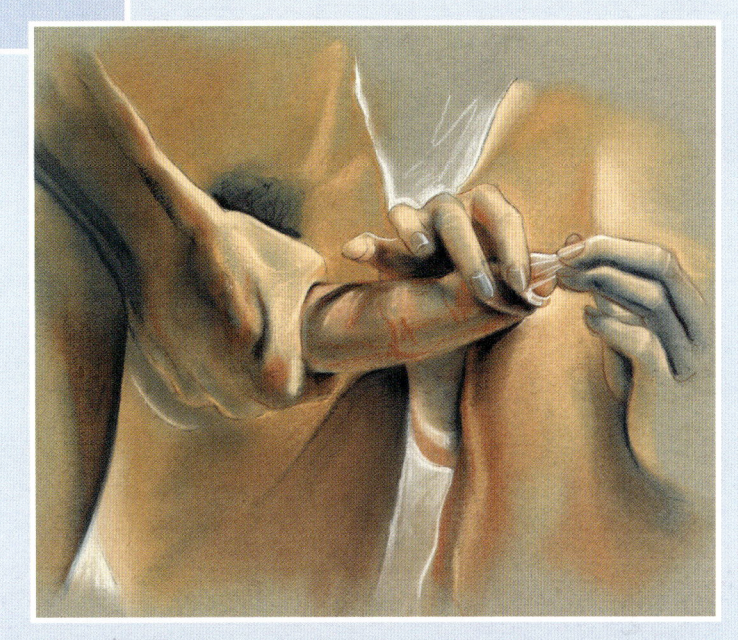

THE CONDOM MUST UNROLL PROPERLY. IF IT GETS STUCK HALF WAY, TEARS OR FEELS TOO TIGHT, IT'S MORE THAN LIKELY THAT HE'S NOT TOO BIG – YOU'VE JUST GOT THE CONDOM INSIDE OUT!

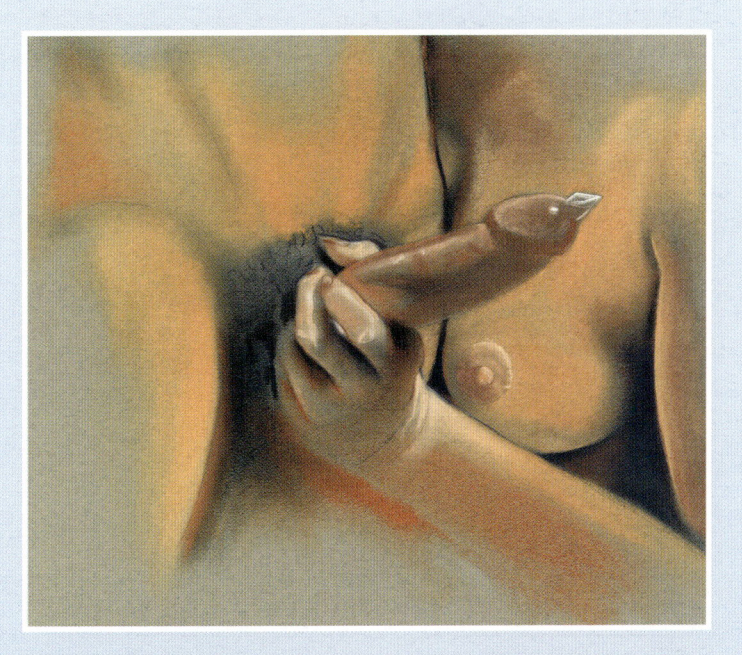

UNROLL THE CONDOM DOWN THE LENGTH OF HIS PENIS, RIGHT TO THE BASE. IF HE GOES SOFT WHILE YOU'RE DOING THIS, GENTLY RUB ROUND THE HEAD OF HIS PENIS WITH THE BALL OF YOUR THUMB

Sexual Positions

Bodies are the same the world over, but we don't all choose to make love in the same way. Ancient and modern sex manuals suggest there are quite a few ways of getting it together with your lover. The *Kama Sutra*, an ancient Hindu work written sometime between 100 and 400 AD, lists eight basic lovemaking positions, and *The Perfumed Garden*, an Arabic treatise written around a thousand years later, suggests eleven. However, each basic posture has literally hundreds of possible variations. One investigator suggested that there are 521 different coital positions, although many of them are only slight variations of the basic forms. Hindu love postures, as described in the *Kama Sutra* and the 15th-century *Ananga Ranga*, have names such as:

Splitting bamboo
Fixing the nail
Pair of tongs

The wheel of Kama
Embrace of crabs
Playing the flute
(for fellatio)

Tiger's tread
(rear entry)
Fluttering and soaring butterfly *(woman on top)*

Ancient Chinese and Hindu texts stressed the importance of perfecting the arts of love

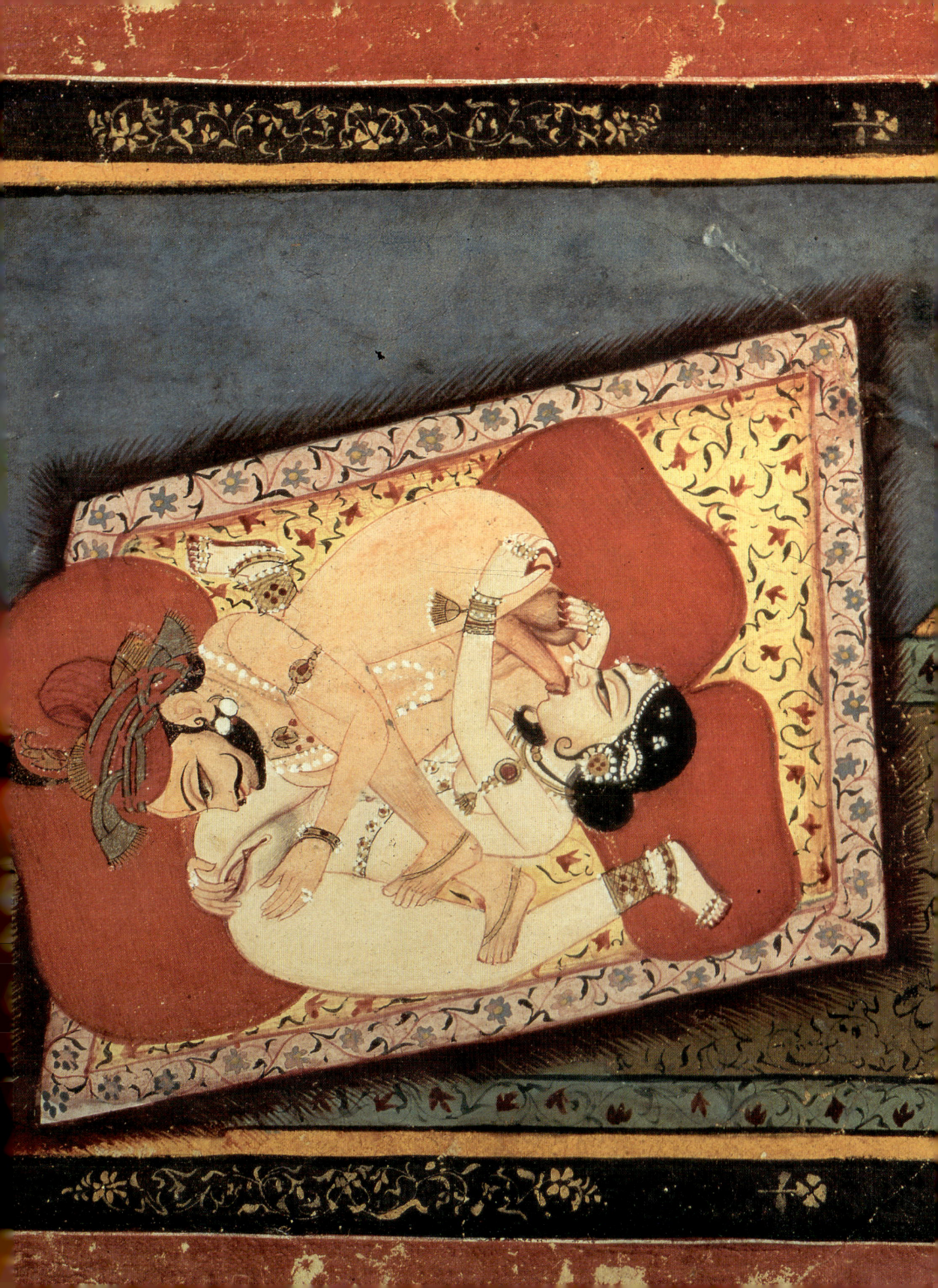

SEXUAL POSITIONS

68

In the *T'ung Hsuan Tzu*, written in the 17th century, the Chinese physician Li T'ung Hsuan describes four basic lovemaking positions and twenty six main variations. He gives the variations delightful names such as "Two fishes side by side", "Flying butterflies", "Cat and mice share a hole", "Leaping wild horses", "Mandarin ducks entwined" and "A phoenix plays in a red cave". His names for the four basic positions are equally poetic:

Close union – *for man on top of woman;*
Unicorn horn – *for woman on man;*
Intimate attachment – *for side by side;*
Sunning fish – *for man entering from the rear.*

How you sit, lie or stand when making love may vary with quite a few factors – your age, your height or weight and your sexual experience. But another important aspect may be the culture you come from. Different societies around the world do seem to favour different sexual positions.

RIGHT: IN THIS REAR-ENTRY POSITION, THE MAN IS FREE TO USE HIS MOUTH ON SENSITIVE AREAS SUCH AS HER EARS AND NECK

BELOW: REAR-ENTRY SEX WHERE YOU LIE "SPOON-FASHION" CAN GIVE YOU BOTH A FEELING OF SPECIAL CLOSENESS

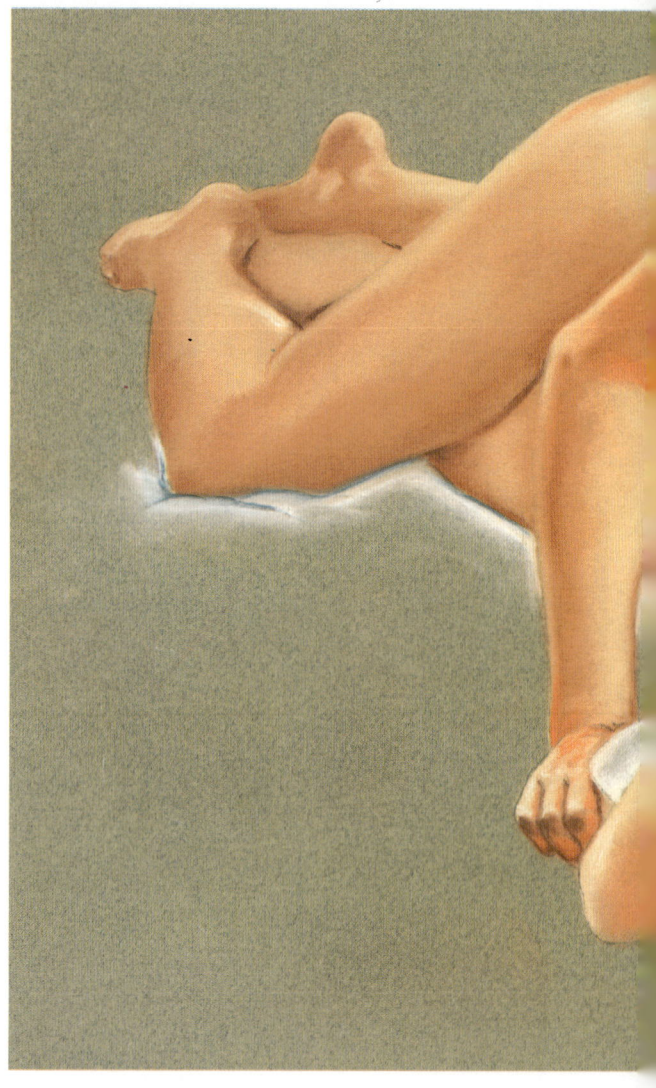

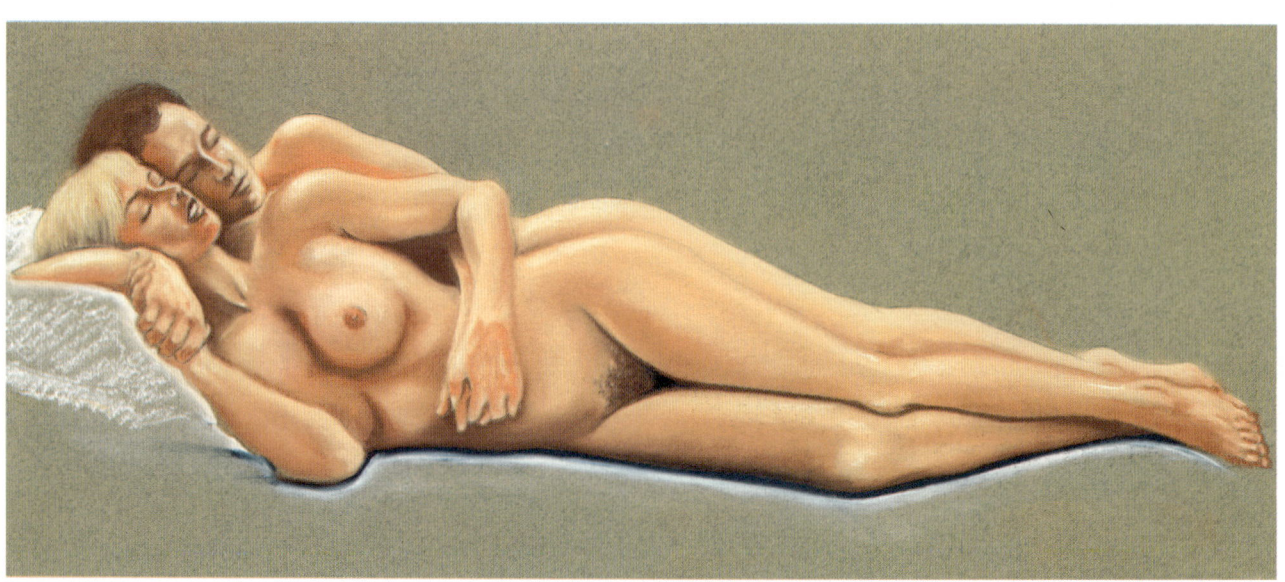

REAR ENTRY

We probably all started off with the same behaviour. Almost all members of the animal kingdom have sex in the rear-entry position, with the female on all fours and the male coming together with her from behind. Cave paintings suggest that our early ancestors had sex in the same way, for very practical reasons. "Doggy fashion" puts the man in a position from which it's reasonably easy to dismount. Since there is no eye contact between the partners, he can have part of his attention on what's going on around them – very handy if you're worried that the odd predatory sabre-toothed tiger or lumbering mammoth might come crashing through the bushes to disturb your pleasure. A new, Western, name for this sexual position is "TV-style", because it allows both partners to keep an eye on the screen while making love!

Rear-entry sexual positions are often favoured in societies where ample buttocks are considered sexy, such as in the Pacific. The Marquesans call it "horse intercourse" and in Arabic it is "after the fashion of a bull". Rear-entry sex is common among the Crow and Hopi nations of North America, the Buka, Kwoma, Marshallese and Wogeo of the Pacific, the Vietnamese and the Lepcha of Asia. Contemporary Russians are also

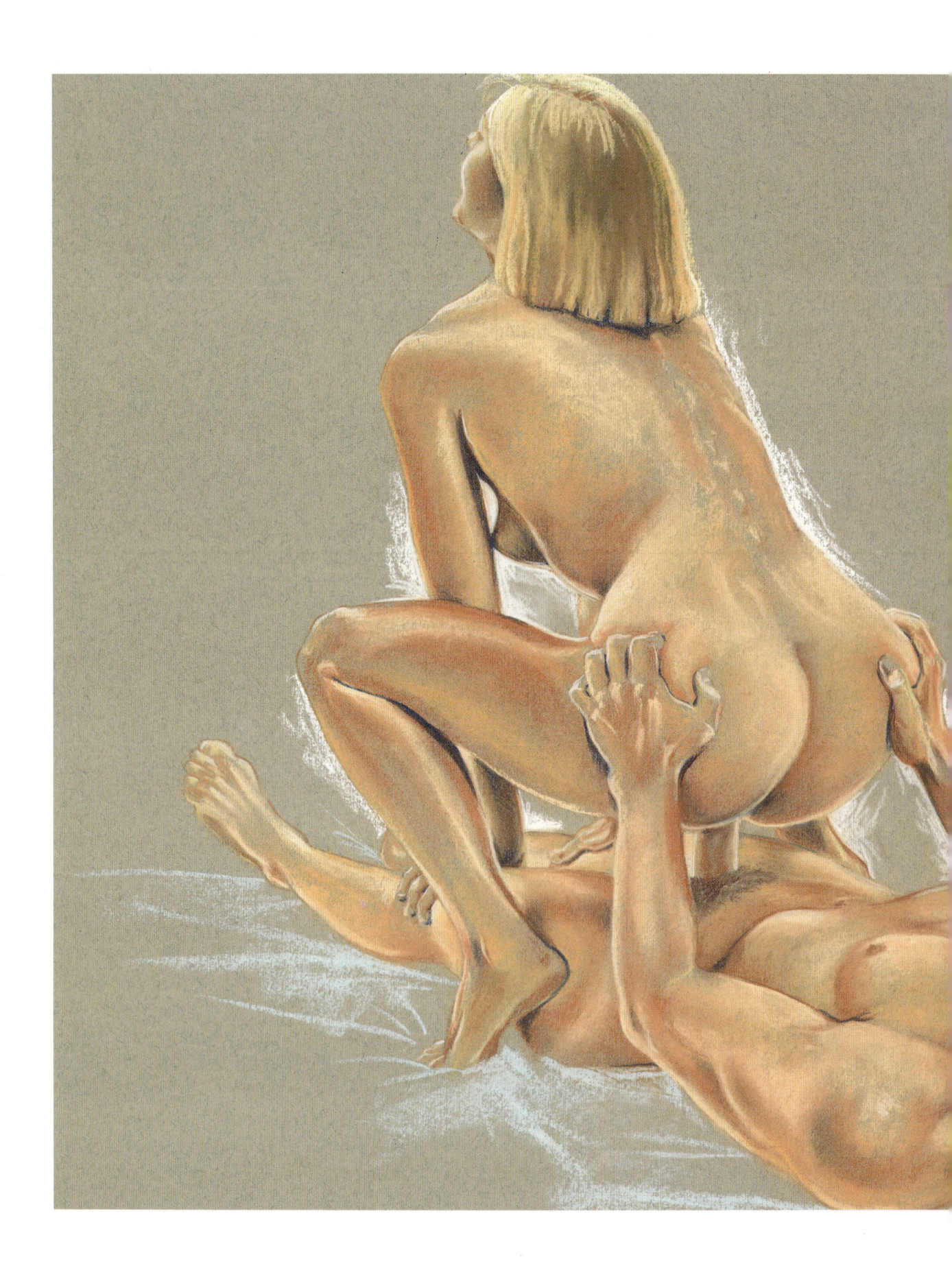

Coming from behind

Try making love "doggy fashion", with the woman lying on her tummy or kneeling. She can lean forward, perhaps over a pillow or over the edge of the bed or a chair. Or he can sit in a chair or lean back against pillows and she can sit in his lap with her back to him. You can also try it standing up, leaning against a chair or table or the bathtub. Many people find this a particularly exciting position, and others find it a shocking one, simply because it reminds them of the way animals have sex. Mind you, our ancestors started out this way, and we are still members of the animal kingdom. Also, this position does allow either or both partners to touch the woman's clitoris and so make sure that she is satisfied.

said to consider it highly erotic, calling it *rakom* or "like a crayfish". One advantage of rear-entry sex done with the couple lying spoon-fashion, is that you can do it under a blanket and you and everyone else can pretend that nothing is going on. Among some native South American peoples, such as the Nambikwara and the Apinaye, rear-entry sex has become their primary sex position for exactly this reason, because it takes place while the community gather together around their shared hearth. British lovers often find doggy sex particularly exciting simply because it is felt to be rather naughty and unusual.

THIS POSITION HAS DISTINCT ADVANTAGES FOR BOTH PARTNERS. IT'S RELAXING FOR HIM, AND GIVES HIM A FULL VIEW OF THE SEXIEST OF SIGHTS – THE FEMALE DERRIERE. AND IT'S GOOD FOR HER BECAUSE SHE IS ABLE TO CONTROL THE ANGLE, SPEED AND DEPTH OF HER PARTNER'S THRUSTS

SEXUAL POSITIONS

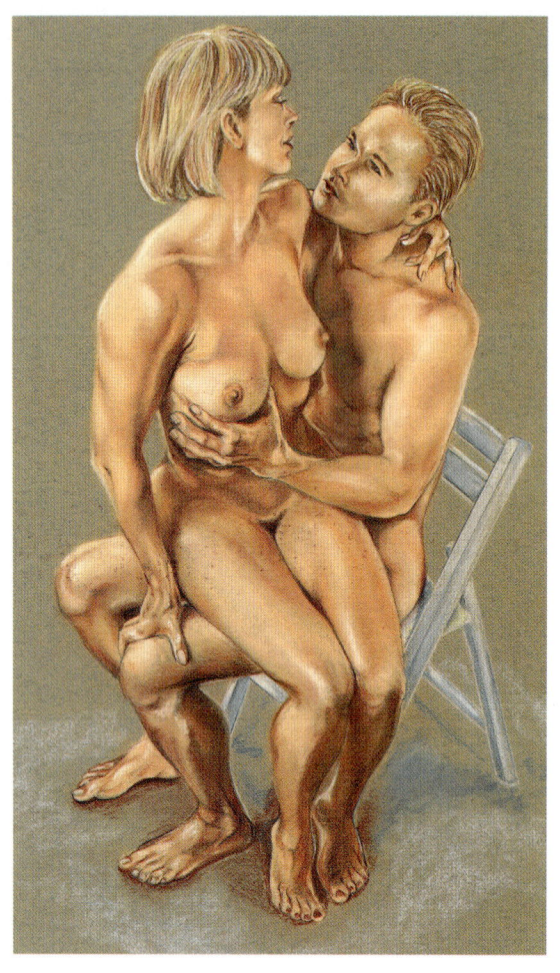

72

HERE, HE CAN EASILY CARESS, LICK AND SUCK HER BREASTS, WHILE SHE HAS TOTAL CONTROL OVER THEIR MOVEMENTS

FACE TO FACE

Face-to-face sex was probably a female invention. It means you can have eye contact, which encouraged the intimate relationship early woman needed to make sure her mate stayed with her instead of hopping off to run after some other female. Face-to-face sex has the advantage of giving the man a view of his partner's breasts. Today, it's the favourite position where breasts are thought to be the most attractive parts of a woman. That usually means societies in the West, where breasts are normally covered up and only seen in the bedroom, and are mainly viewed in sexual terms rather than for breastfeeding babies.

MAN ON TOP

In many cultures, one particular sexual position is seen as "the correct way" of doing it. The "missionary" position is the one most frequently used by couples in the United States, Japan, Britain and the Westernized parts of South America. It's often considered the only proper, acceptable way of making love and is so-named, it is said, because Pacific islanders saw missionaries making love and were amused that they stuck to this one decorous position. In Tuscany, it's known as the "angelic position", but some Arabic-speaking groups call it the "manner of serpents".

For missionary-style sex, the man lies on top and in between the legs of his partner, supporting himself on his elbows. The problem with this position is that it can be quite limiting for both partners. If the man is not to lean heavily on the woman, he has to keep both hands or elbows down, which means he cannot caress her breasts or her clitoris or other parts with ease. His penis can receive all the stimulation it needs from the in-and-out motion, which is well under his control in this position, but his partner may find that the speed, thrust and angle of penetration simply does not excite or satisfy her.

A variation on man on top is the "Oceanic" position, found in the islands of the Pacific, although many societies in Africa, Asia and South America use it too. In this, the woman lies on her back as the man squats or kneels between her legs. By not having to balance on his arms, the man is free to caress his partner and so make sure she is as sexually satisfied as he is. According to the Trobriand Islanders of Papua New Guinea, one advantage of the Oceanic position is that it can be carried out with as little body contact as possible,

WITH THE MAN ON TOP, A COUPLE CAN VARY THE PRESSURE HE PLACES ON HER. SOME WOMEN FIND IT PARTICULARLY EXCITING TO HAVE THEIR MAN PRESSING DOWN HEAVILY BETWEEN THEIR LEGS

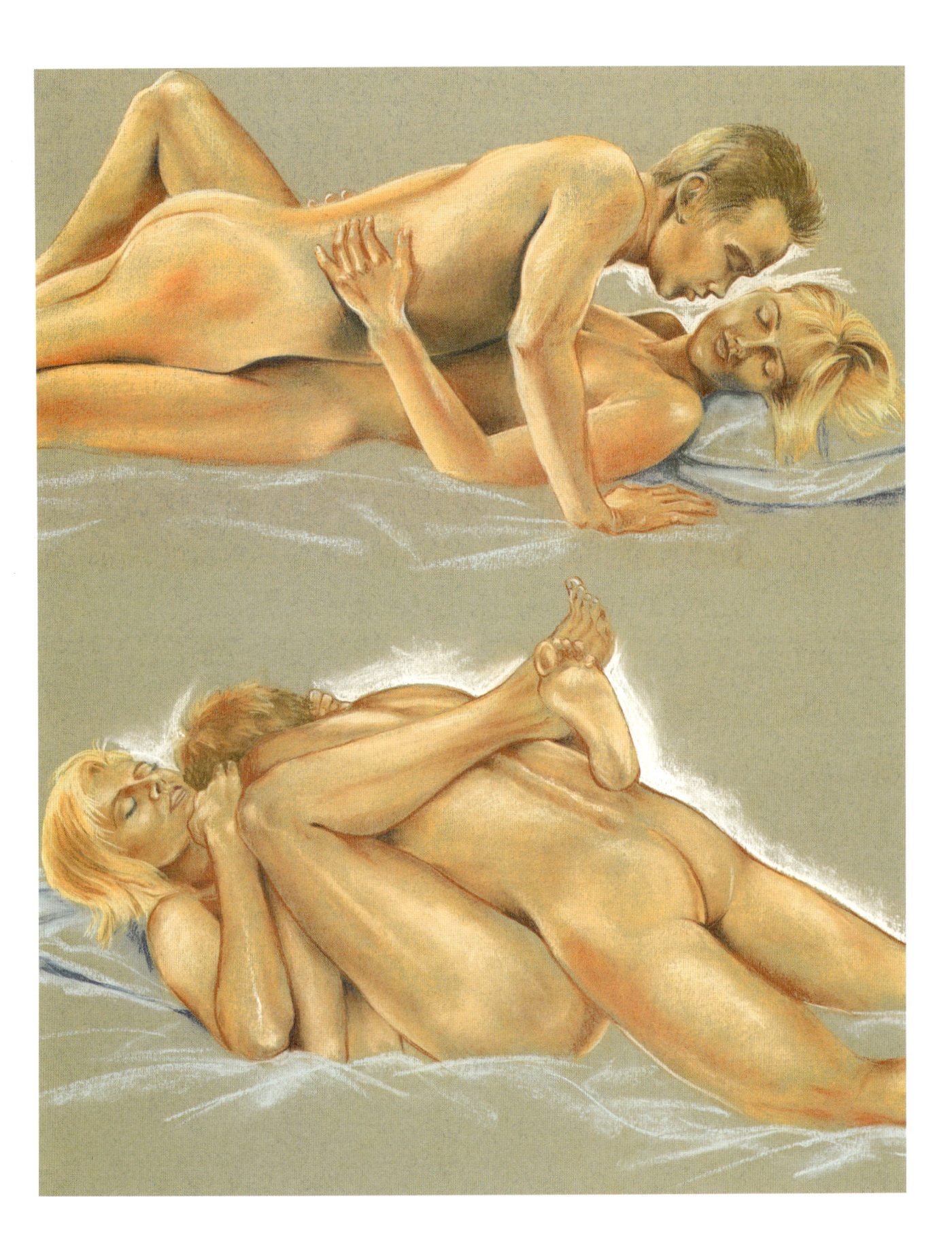

so a woman married to an old or ugly man can keep as far away from him as possible. The Tallensi of Africa mention another advantage – with the man squatting in a rather awkward position, it means that once she's had her fill, all the woman needs to do is nudge him with her knee and he falls over!

The *Ananga Ranga*, which describes positions still used in Asia, as well as around the globe, lists several variations on this, depending on whether the woman raises her legs and rests her knees on the man's chest or stretches them across his shoulders, or wraps them around his back. She can also remain with her hips on the bed or raise them and rest on his thighs. He can lean back, only touching her with his hands and by genital contact. Or, if the couple want to take full advantage of this position, he can lean over, gathering her in his arms.

IF HER LEGS ARE STRETCHED OVER HIS SHOULDERS, HE CAN PENETRATE DEEPLY AND SHE HAS A SURPRISING AMOUNT OF MOVEMENT

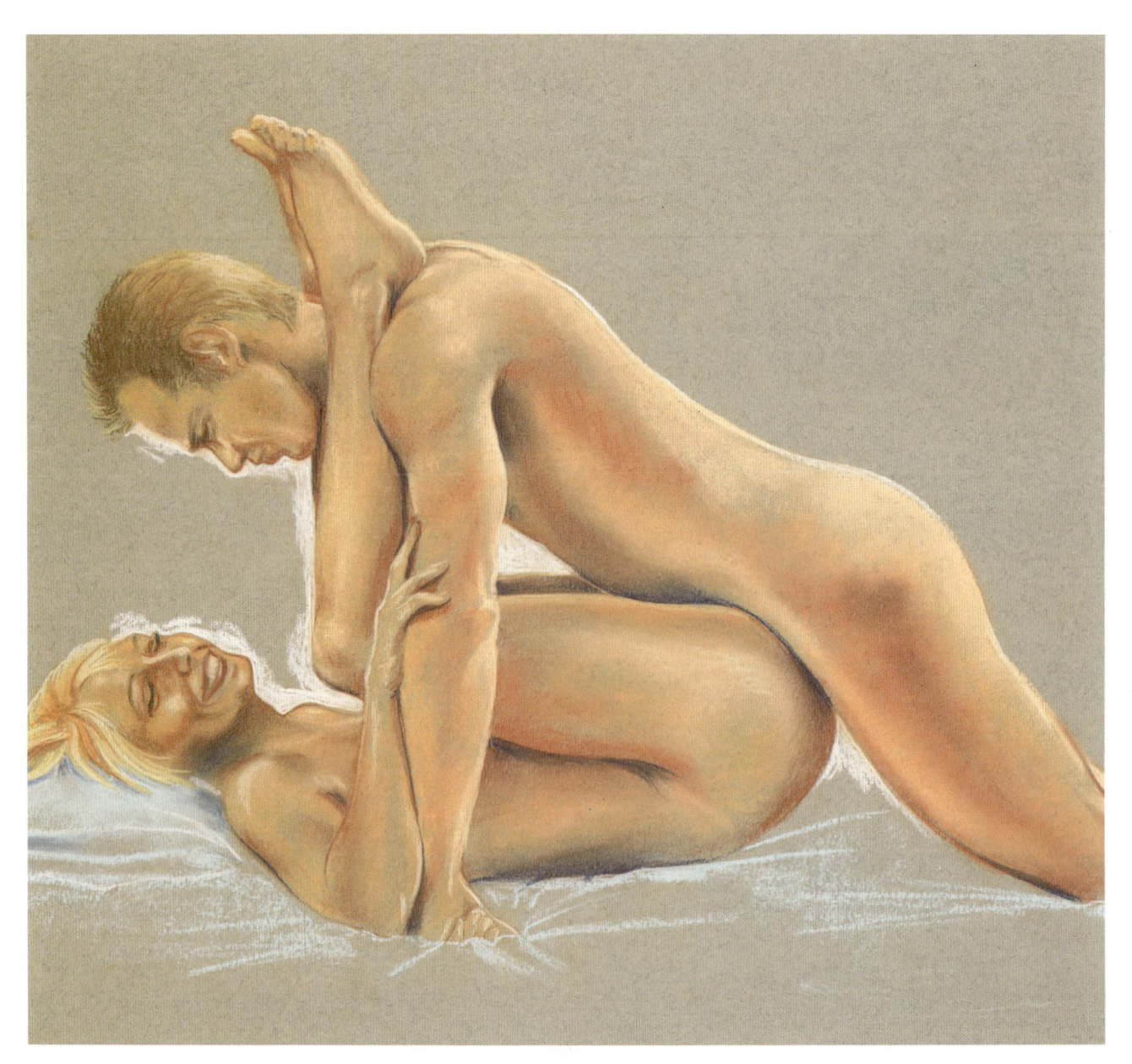

Ancient wisdom

As we discovered in Chapter 1, the *Kama Sutra* describes men and women as belonging to a certain sexual class. According to the size of their penes, men are Hares, Bulls or Horses and, based on the depth of their vaginas, women are Deer, Mares or Elephants. It also suggests that there are six equal and nine unequal types of sexual union.

But the *Kama Sutra* doesn't rule out sexual satisfaction if a Hare man has sex with an Elephant woman, or a Horse with a Deer – it's just that extra care and special positions may be advisable. It is recommended that the Deer should try sex in ways that widen her vagina. One is to lie with her head lower than her hips, perhaps supporting her buttocks on a cushion, and to use oil or lotion to make penetration easier. Another is to bend her knees, keeping her feet on the ground, in the "yawning position". Yet another is the "Indrani position", where the legs are doubled up and the hips slightly raised.

Elephant women, according to the *Kama Sutra*, use the "clasping position", the "pressing position", the "twining position" and the "Mare's position". In the "clasping position", the couple can lie side by side or one on top of the other, but in all cases the legs are stretched straight out. If she presses him with her thighs, that is the "pressing position". If she wraps one of her thighs over him, that is the "twining position". And if she can squeeze his penis with the muscles of her vagina, that is the "Mare's position"!

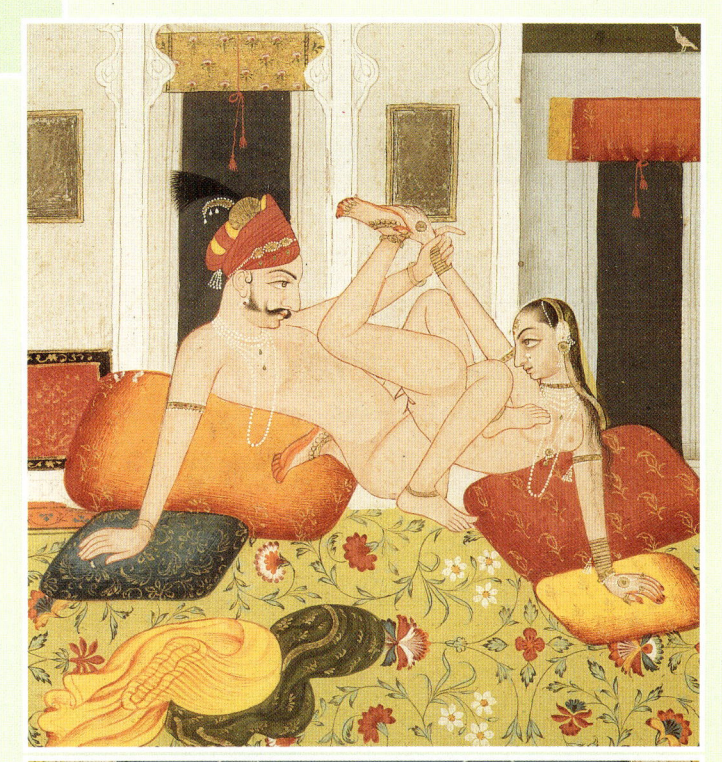

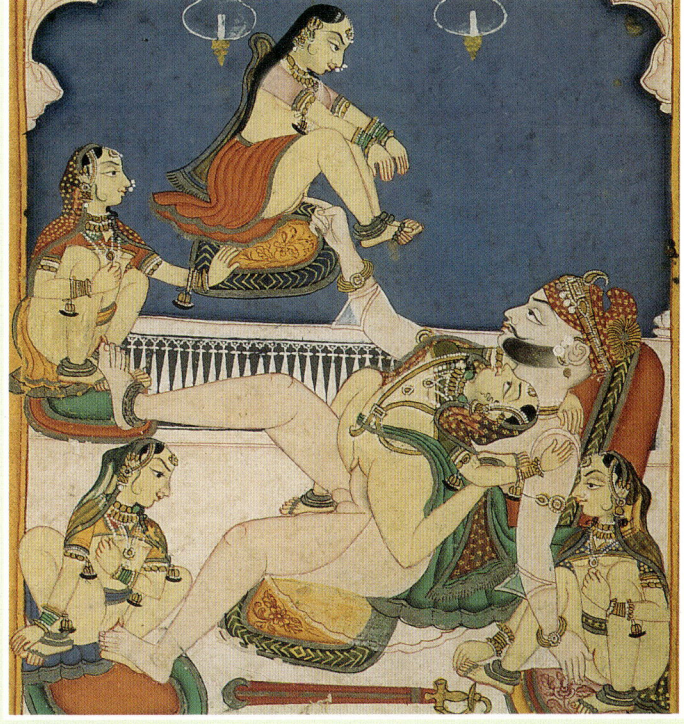

THE *KAMA SUTRA* ENCOURAGES COUPLES WHO HAVE DIFFICULTY GETTING IT TOGETHER TO EXPERIMENT AS MUCH AS POSSIBLE

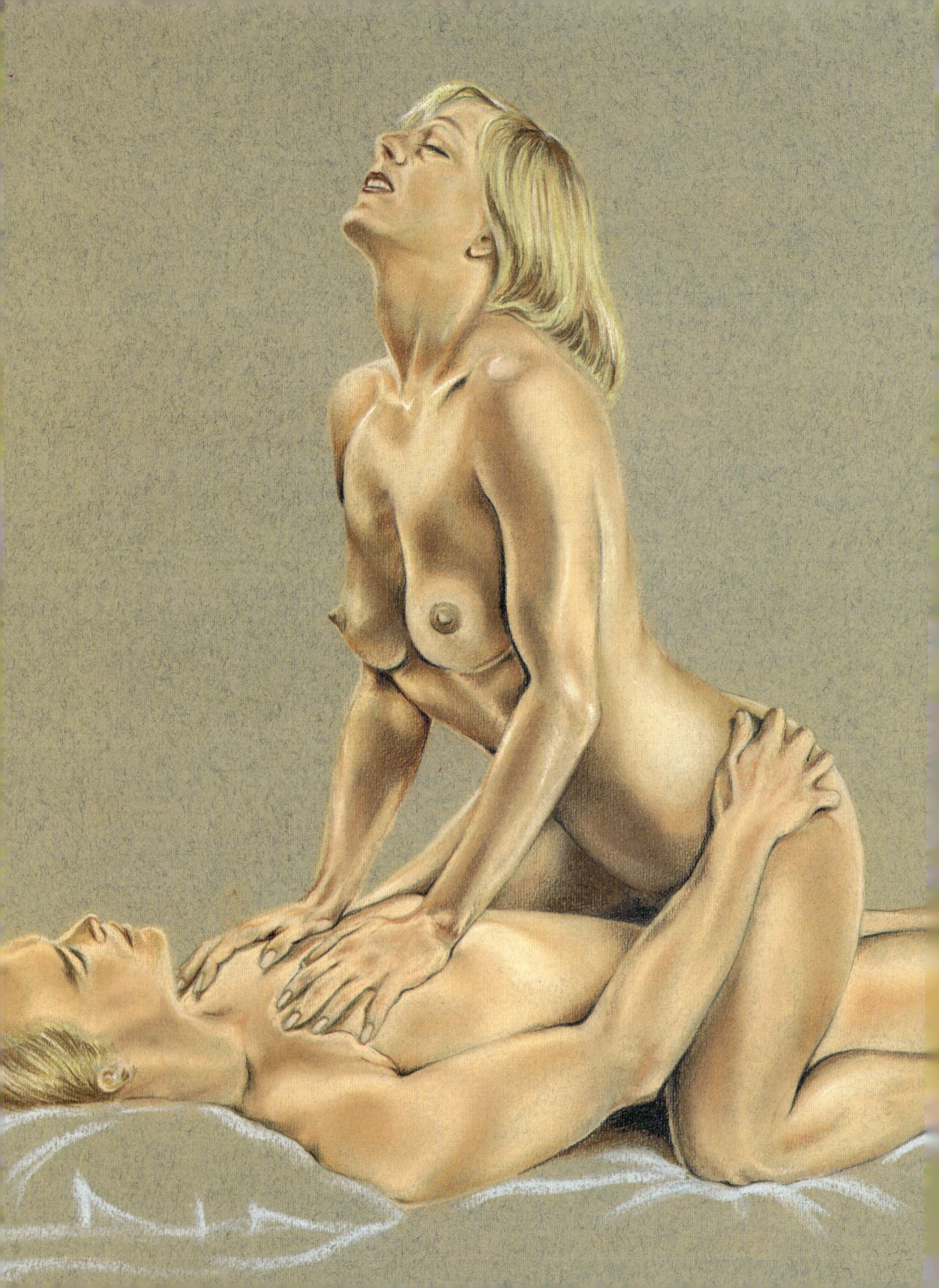

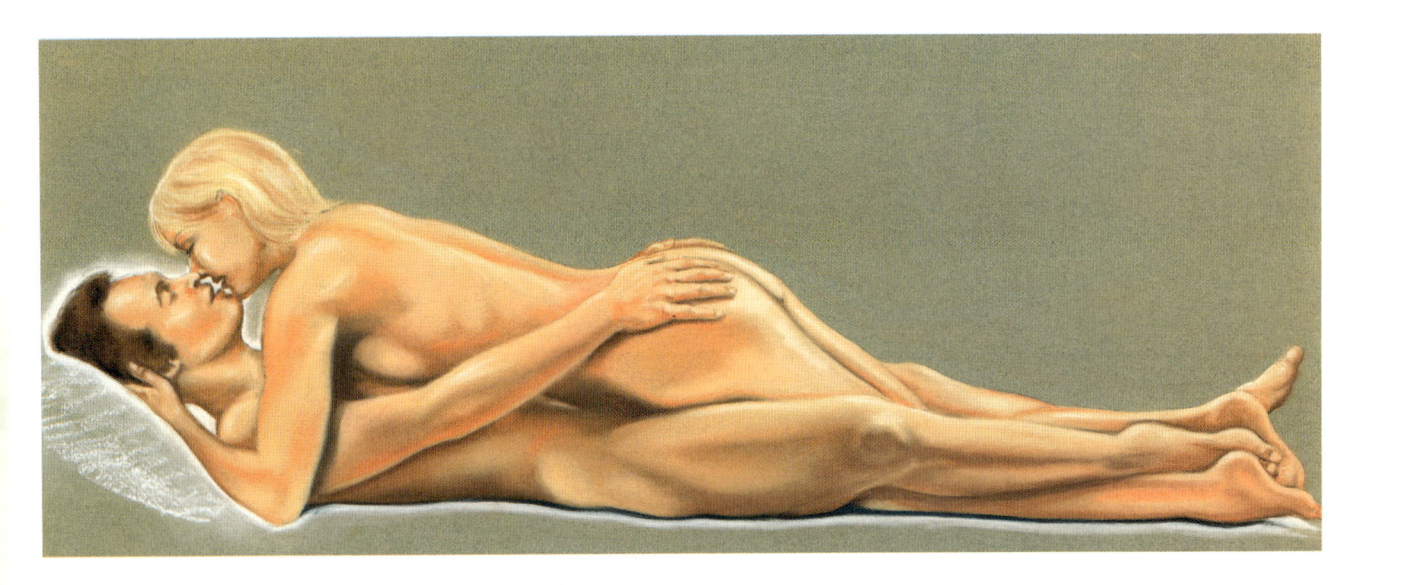

Give it a go!

If you've never tried woman on top, try it tonight with your partner. You can lie chest to chest, kissing and using your tongues and teeth on each other. Or, she can kneel upright while both of you allow your hands free rein over each other's body. Either way, you may find that making love in this position gives your lovemaking a totally new dimension!

WOMAN ON TOP

Cultural groups across most of the South Pacific isles prefer the woman to be on top during lovemaking, but the woman-on-top sexual position is greatly frowned on in societies where male dominance is felt to be particularly important, or where female dominance is seen to be rather frightening. The Native American Navaho actually believe that a man can become pregnant if he has sex with a woman in this position, but the Crow and Hopi nations are happy to indulge, as are the Murngin people of Australia.

In this position, the woman lies on top of her partner, either with both legs astride his, or with one or both legs inside his thighs. He may be able to take her weight on his chest, allowing her to have one or both hands free to caress him thoroughly or to guide his hands.

A woman may well discover that she climaxes much more easily in this position. Not only can she decide the angle and set the pace of the movement, but she will probably find that this is the ideal position for clitoral stimulation. Another advantage is that the man can have his hands entirely free to stroke and hold her, and to touch her breasts or clitoris. Many men also get a special enjoyment from this position. Because they find it less tiring, it often allows them to last much longer and to enjoy lovemaking more.

ABOVE: WITH HER LEGS INSIDE HIS, THIS POSITION DOES NOT ALLOW FOR DEEP PENETRATION, BUT IT MAKES UP FOR THAT IN CLITORAL STIMULATION

OPPOSITE: WOMAN ON TOP MAY BE THE BEST POSITION FOR THE WOMAN. IT PUTS HER IN CHARGE AND LETS HER MAKE SURE SHE REACHES A SATISFYING CLIMAX

SEXUAL POSITIONS

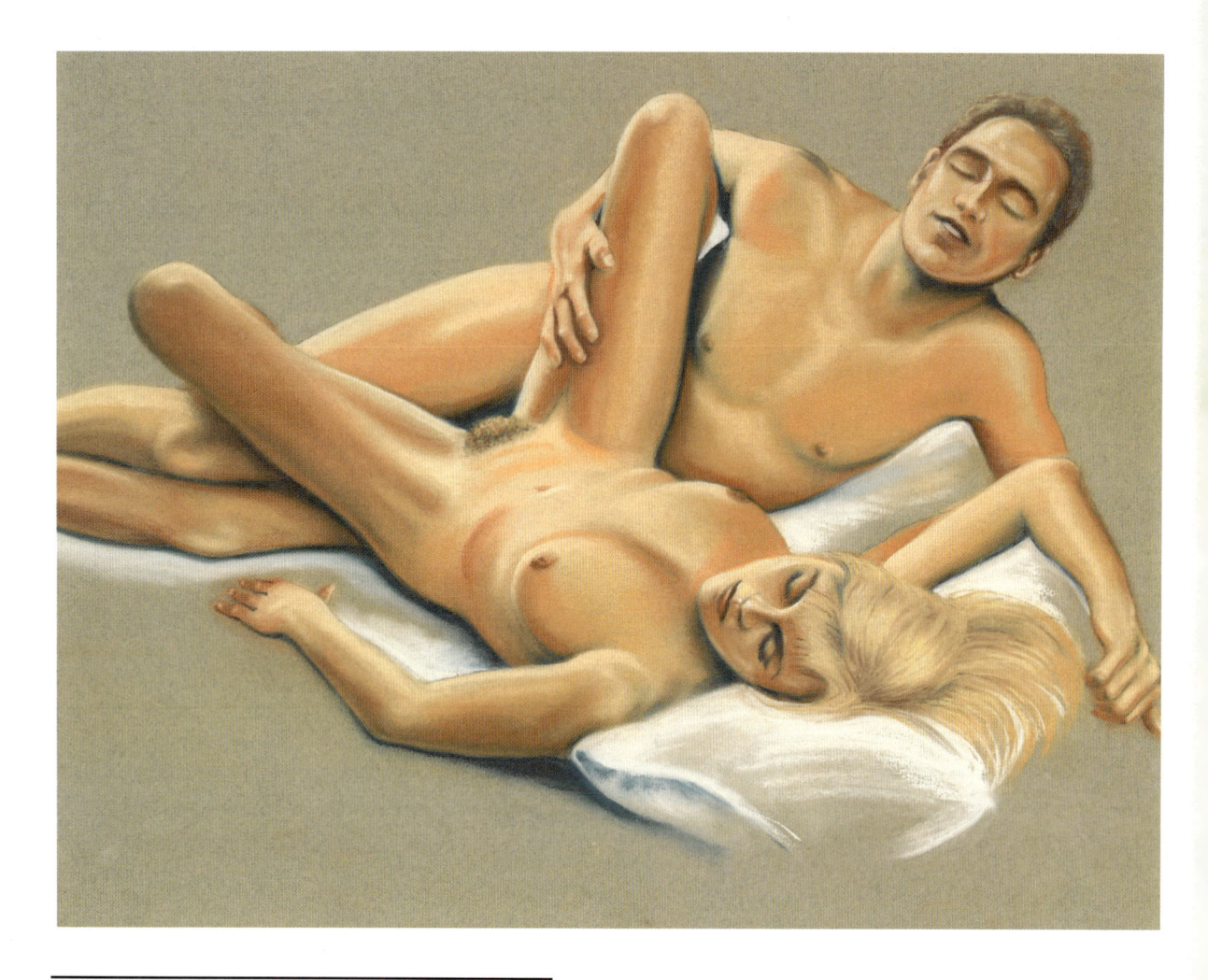

SIDE BY SIDE

Both the Bala from Zaire and the Tikopia, who live on an island in the Pacific, believe that the best lovemaking position is side by side. In this, both partners lie down face to face, on their sides. The Marquesana have named this the "gecko lizard manner", and it's also the favoured position in many African societies, such as the Masai, the Tiswana, the Dogon and the Bambara.

Some people can find it quite difficult to enter properly in the side-by-side position, a difficulty found particularly by the Tikopia, since they have a taboo against touching either their own or their partner's genitals. Sex among the Tikopia has to be strictly a "Look Ma, no hands!" affair.

ABOVE: THIS GIVES LOVERS THE CHANCE TO CARESS EACH OTHER TO THE FULL, AND SEE WHAT EFFECT THIS IS HAVING

RIGHT: STANDING SEX CAN BROADEN YOUR REPERTOIRE, BUT YOU MAY NEED TO BE FIT AND STRONG TO HOLD THIS KIND OF POSITION

On the side

If you want to try the side-by-side position, you might like to start off with one or the other on top and then roll over. You also need to hold on and move together or you might lose touch. It makes for long, slow, gentle and loving sex, with both of you able to touch and hold to your hearts' content.

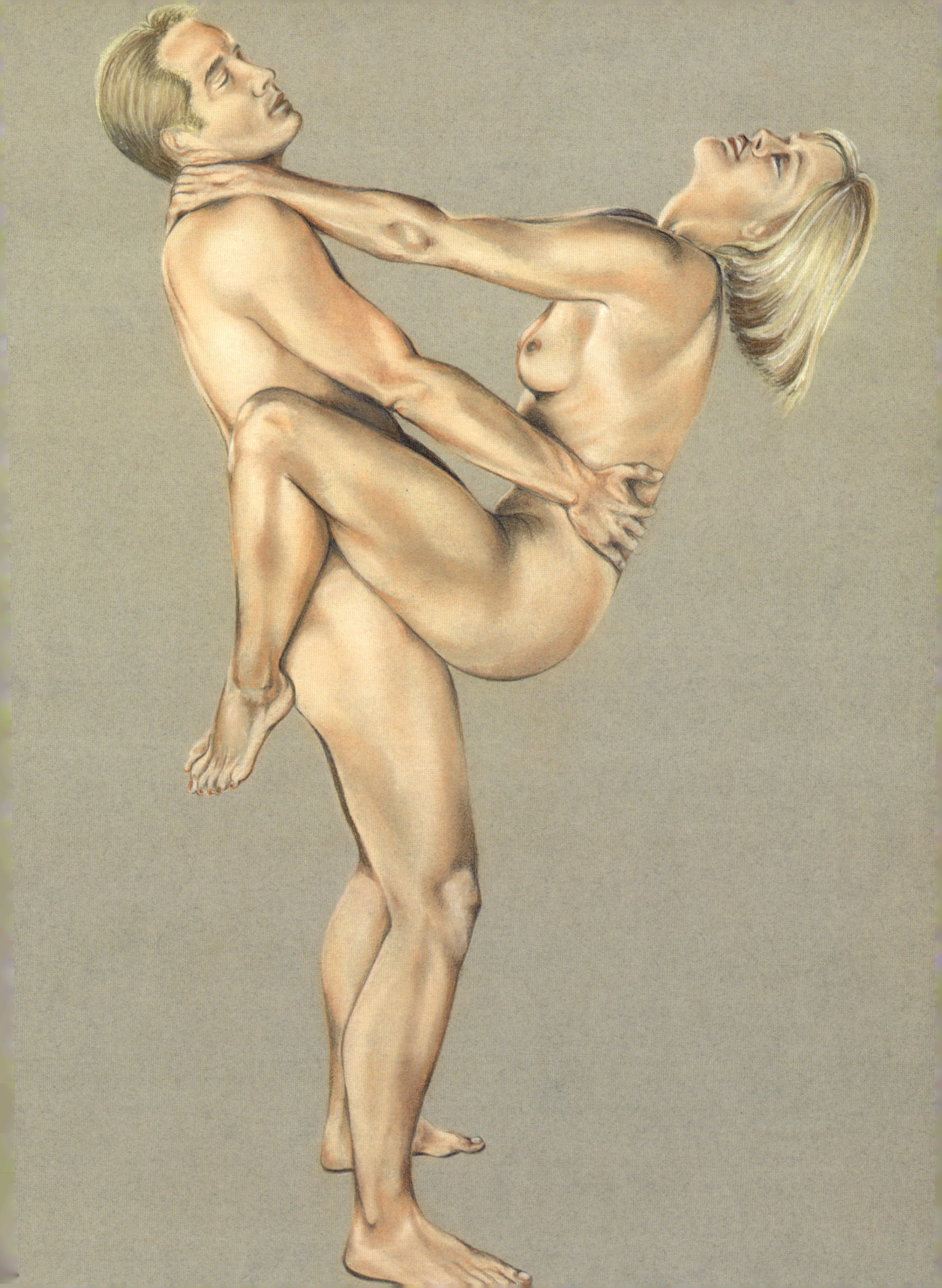

STANDING UP

In the *Kama Sutra*, positions that allow you to make love standing up are called "supported" or "suspended" congress. In *The Perfumed Garden*, they are given the more imaginative titles "belly to belly" and "driving the peg home". Not surprisingly, nobody seems to pick them as first choice for general sex as they are a quite tiring and difficult way of making love. The Fijians reserve standing positions entirely for premarital or extramarital affairs. They are exceptionally good, however, for fun in the shower or if you are caught by passion away from the bedroom. If one of you is much shorter than the other, you might need a footstool, or the lighter partner can hop up and wrap their legs round the taller, heavier partner's thighs, while being held up by the bottom or thighs.

SITTING DOWN

In the mountainous islands of the central Pacific, the Marquesans have seated sex with the woman astride her partner's lap. Native Australians opt for sitting positions, too. The man sits on the ground, in a chair or on a bed, and the woman sits in his lap with her legs astride his. This position, like woman on top, gives her control and him staying power, and allows him to use his tongue or lips on her breasts. Among the Yapese, who live on an island in the Carolines, couples favour a seated position with the woman facing and squatting on top of her seated partner. A further twist is that Yapese women believe that orgasm is better if they make love on a full bladder and can pass water at the moment of climax.

SEX IN PREGNANCY

Sex during pregnancy can be a joy, but it does need some thought beforehand. Tender breasts and a bump can make sex in your usual positions unpleasant or painful. If you generally make love in the man-on-top "missionary" position, it's time to move to woman on top, because it doesn't press

Singin' in the rain

Try standing-up love in the shower. Set the temperature to a sexy sizzle, and slather plenty of soap over each other to help your hands glide over your lover's body with maximum ease. But – take care not to slip!

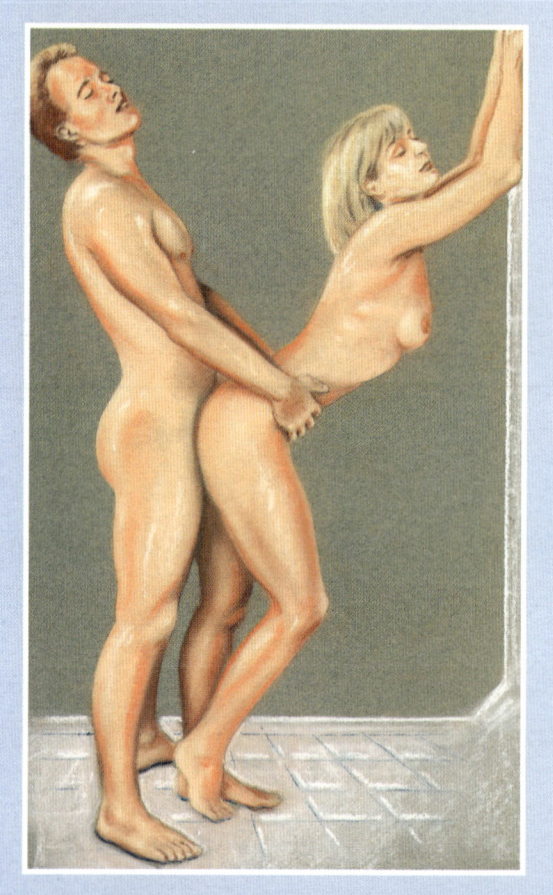

SEX ON YOUR FEET MAY BE TIRING, BUT IT COULD BE WELL WORTH IT. TAKING HIS PARTNER FROM THE REAR, A STANDING LOVER HAS EVERY OPPORTUNITY TO TOUCH HER BREASTS AND CLITORIS AND SO MAKE SURE SHE RECEIVES AS MUCH PLEASURE AS HE DOES

RIGHT: SITTING THIS ONE OUT NEEDN'T MEAN MISSING ANY OF THE FUN. THIS IS ANOTHER POSITION WHERE THE MAN CAN USE HIS HANDS TO FULL, STIMULATING EFFECT

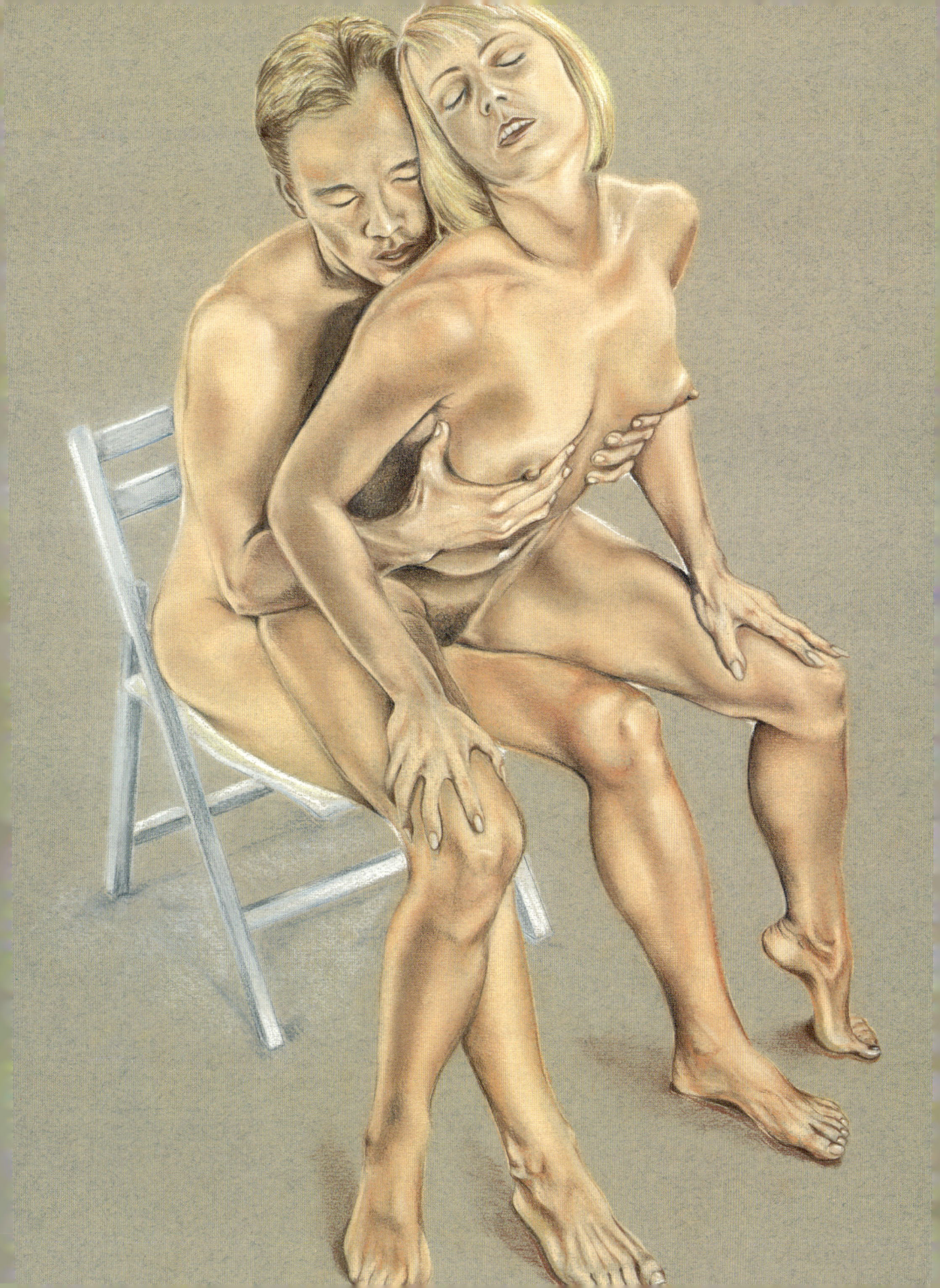

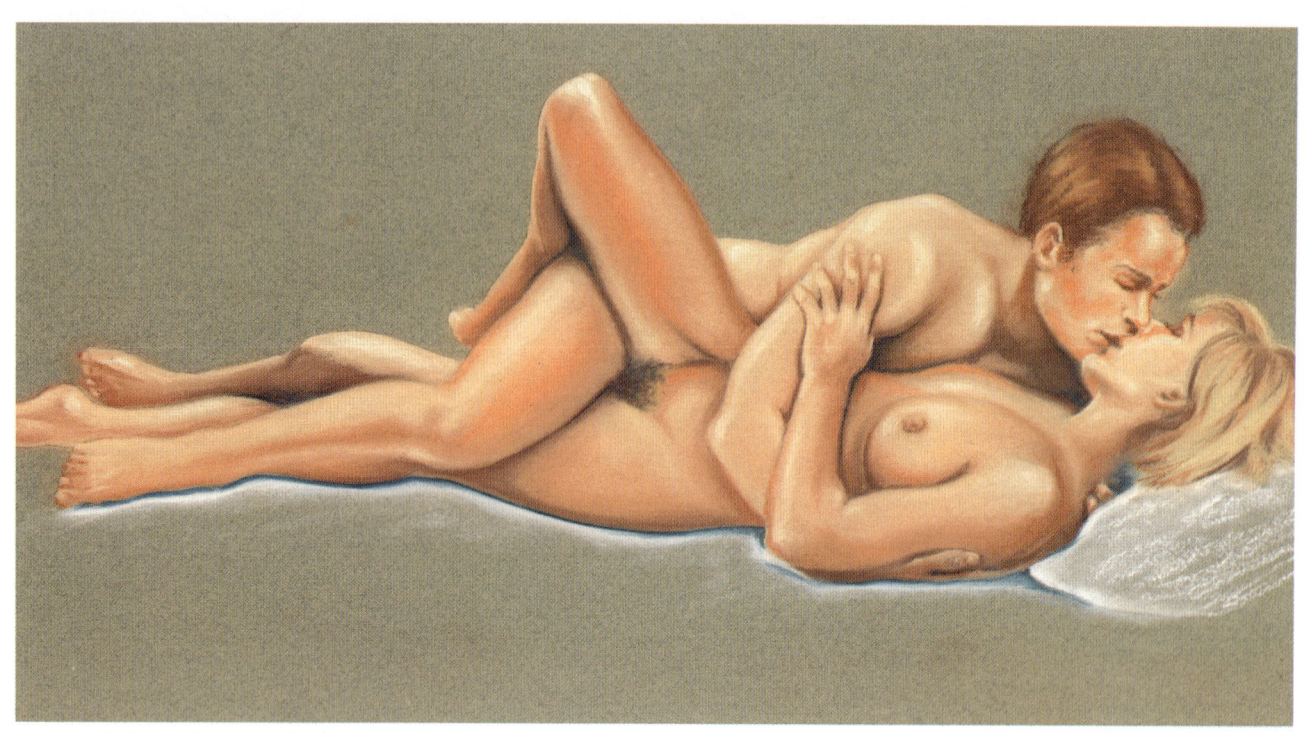

so hard on delicate places. As the pregnancy progresses, when the baby's growing bulk literally comes between you, you will find that "scissors" positions, with the man lying half on and half off his partner, or side-by-side rear entry, will make sex easier and more comfortable. Above all, remember that lovemaking does not always have to mean full intercourse. Kissing, cuddling or exploring other ways of touching can be just as powerful in giving you both the pleasure and reassurance you need at this time.

For the first few months after the birth, you may find that positions and love-play that were once exciting and pleasant have become uncomfortable or painful. You may find lovemaking is best when the woman is on top. She can then control the angle and strength of coital thrusts and so make sure that tender flesh is not bruised and scar tissue not stressed. For some time after birth, the male partner should take special care to be sensitive to the woman's reactions while making love, so as to make sure that it is satisfaction and not pain that she is getting from their love-play. If he hasn't been in the habit of watching, listening and responding to her

LYING FACE TO FACE WITH THE MAN ON TOP DOESN'T HAVE TO BE EXACTLY THE SAME EACH AND EVERY TIME. TRY TWINING YOUR LEGS TOGETHER IN ALL KINDS OF POSITIONS TO GIVE YOUR LOVING SOMETHING OF A DIFFERENT FLAVOUR

every reaction before, he may well find that getting used to doing so at this time can transform a so-so love-life into a no-holds-barred fireworks display!

Ringing the changes

You can ring eternal changes to sex positions by bending or straightening legs, sitting up, leaning over, or using pillows, chairs or tables to assist you. People all over the world make love in hundreds of different ways. Why not celebrate your membership of the Global Village by trying something new today? You don't have to tie yourself in knots, but neither do you have to lie still and keep doing it the same way. Experiment and see what tickles your fancy.

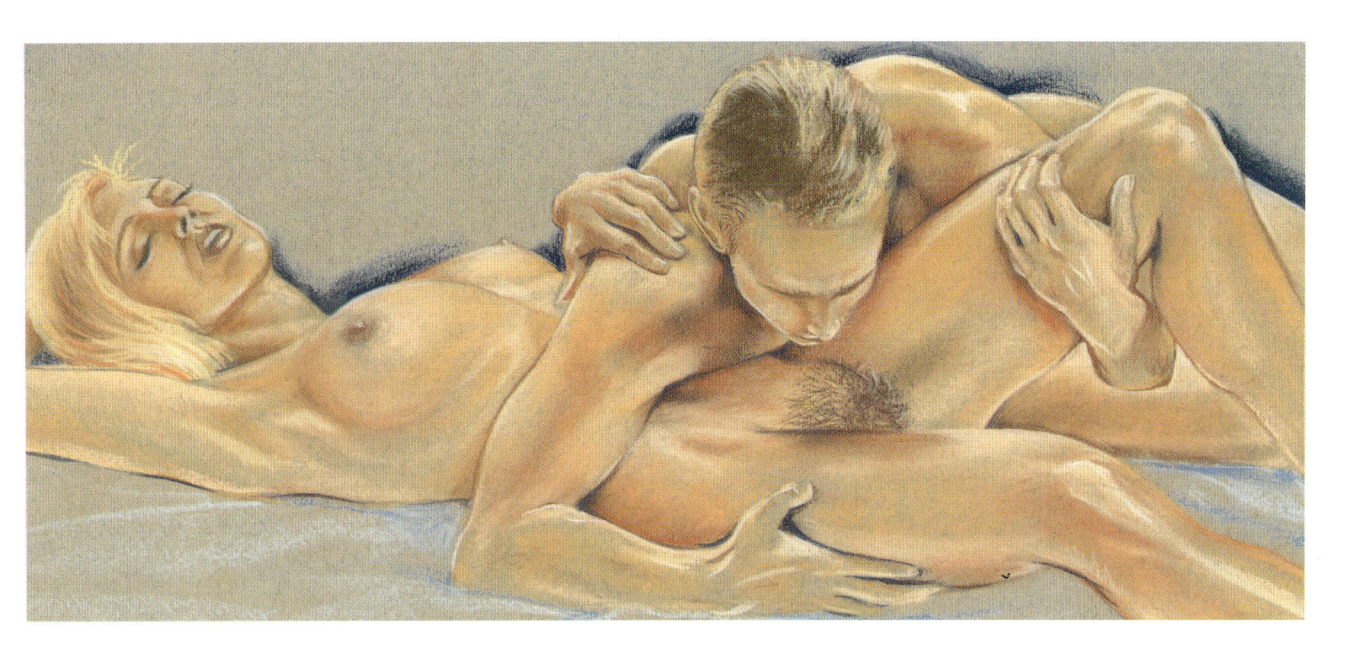

Oral sex

Many people are turned on by the sight, taste and smell of their partner's genitals. They find that oral sex, where you use your mouth on those very private parts, is not only physically pleasant, but it is the perfect way of showing just how tasty you think your partner is.

This isn't true in every society. Among the Fang, for instance, oral sex by either husband or wife would be considered as good grounds for a divorce, and the Ila think any mouth-to-genital contact is downright criminal! But oral sex is favoured by many cultural groups, especially those in the Pacific. Mutual oral sex figures in the sexual techniques that Mangaian teenagers learn as part of their education for adult lfe.

Some people prefer gentle licking, when being mouthed by their lover. You can find out what your partner likes by gently running your tongue and lips round their genitals. Others like the attention to be firmer, with the glans or clitoris being sucked and even gently nipped. In spite of the term "blow job" don't, ever, be tempted to blow into the opening at the end of his penis or into her vagina. You could give your partner a really nasty infection or even an embolism.

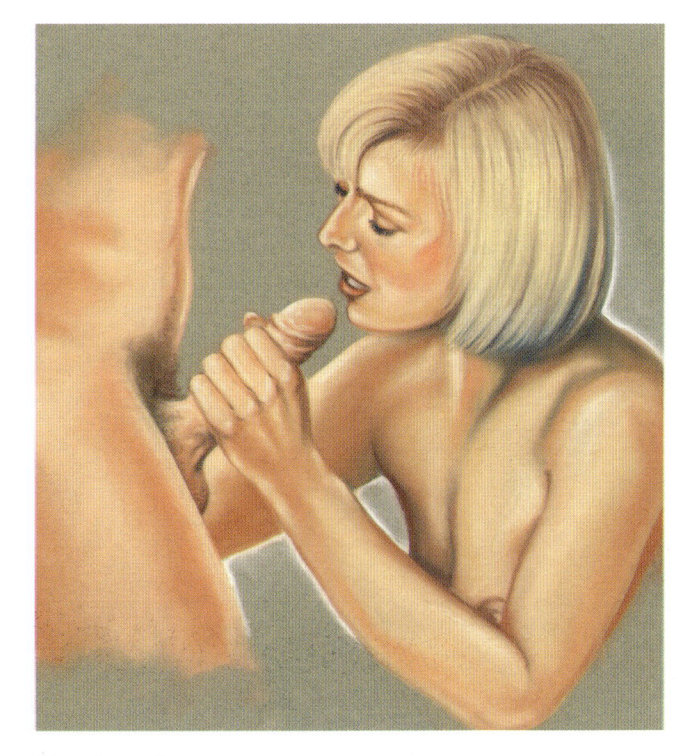

Top: A man's tongue can often give extremely sensitive stimulation

Above: Many men particularly enjoy gentle sucking and having a tongue run around the glans

Over Page: It doesn't take that much ingenuity to find a position where you can enjoy mutual oral stimulation

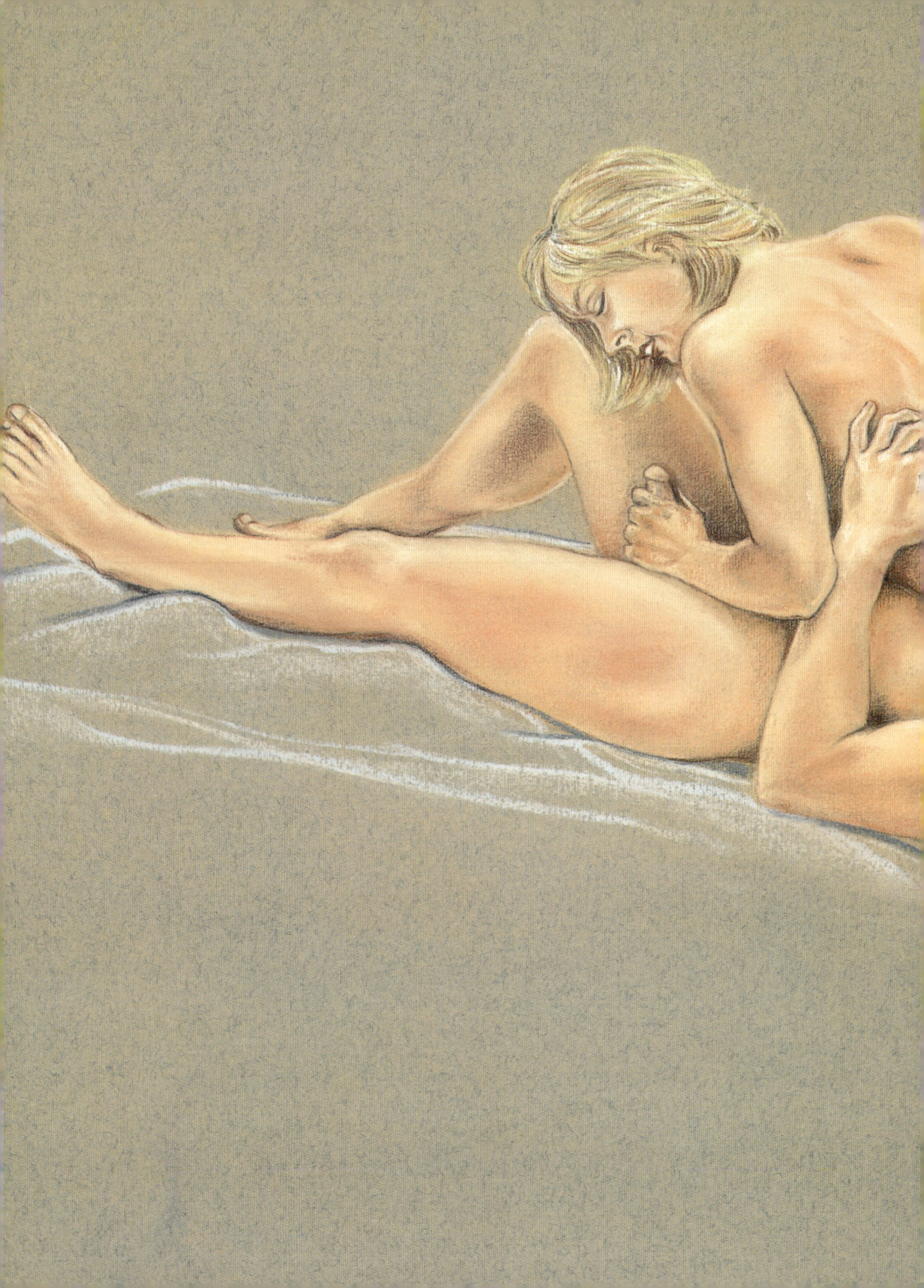

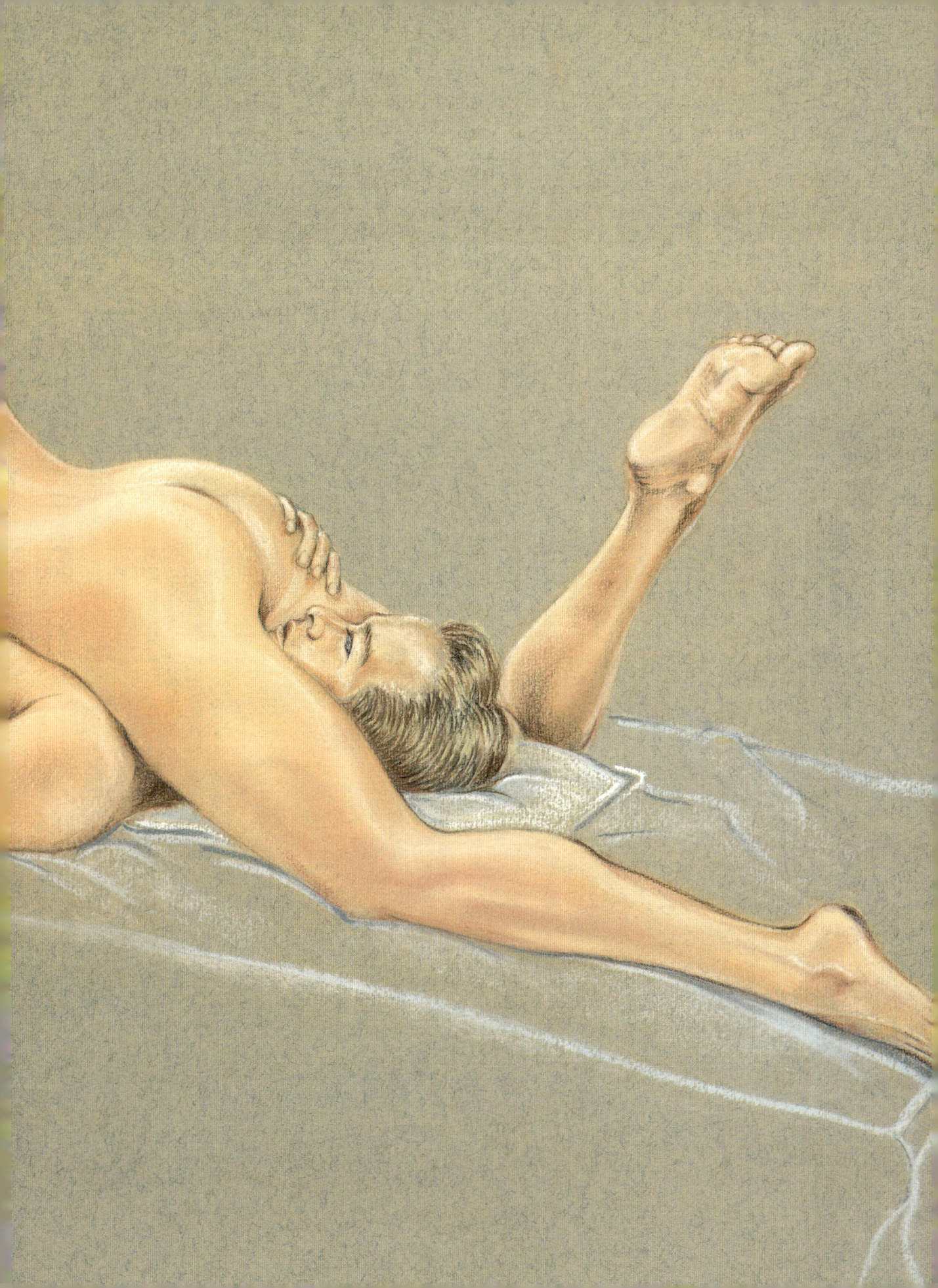

A PLACE AND A TIME

In the West, we tend to feel that sex is a pastime that should be kept to the bedroom, a view that certainly isn't shared by everyone on this planet. As mentioned in Chapter 3, the Yucatec and Mayans of South America might agree with the Western viewpoint, to the point of having a total taboo against sex outdoors, but in Papua New Guinea, there is a taboo against having sex indoors. The Yapese, from the Carolines, the Aluetians and the Formosans, all make love in the open air, and privacy is no big thing, either, in these cultures. Quite a few of the societies in Oceania, such as The Yapese, Trukese and Trobrianders, make love in public as a part of erotic and ceremonial festivals. There is also very little privacy in societies where whole families or communities share sleeping and living quarters. In Polynesia, couples will make love without worrying that there are others in the same room, asleep, pretending to be asleep, or also engaged in lovemaking!

The place...

You could try making love in a lift, car, restaurant or a train – you name it and someone is bound to have tried it before you. If your behaviour is not offensive to anyone else, that is, remaining private even though it is in a public place, then you are harming no one. If you are seen, however, in most societies you could be had up for a range of offences, so do be discreet and careful.

Perhaps the ultimate in risky, exhibitionist behaviour is the so-called "Mile High" Club, where you become a "member" if you make love in a plane. However, the captain has the right to land at the nearest airport and throw you off if your behaviour is upsetting other passengers. This has certainly been done to passengers who refused to put out cigarettes or who were drunk and disorderly. And the airline has the right to bill you for the entire cost of such a detour, so your sexual adventure could be ruinously expensive. It might actually be cheaper to rent a small plane or helicopter for a private "fly by". Many firms now offer trips in hot air balloons and other flying machines, for that very "special" occasion. Just how special do you want it to be!

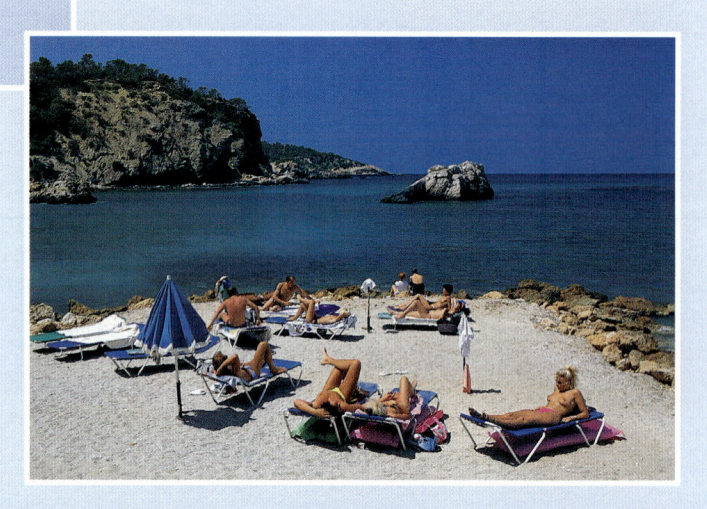

WHY NOT TRY SOME "AL FRESCO" SEX WHEN YOU ARE NEXT HAVING A RELAXING BREAK IN A SUNNY SPOT – BUT BE DISCREET!

The time...

Many Westerners often feel that the proper, discreet time to make love is at night, under cover of darkness, but not for the same reasons as the people of certain other cultures. The Fang, an African society, believe that making love during the daytime will lead to ill-health. And among the African Zulu, daytime sex is considered fit only for beasts, not human beings.

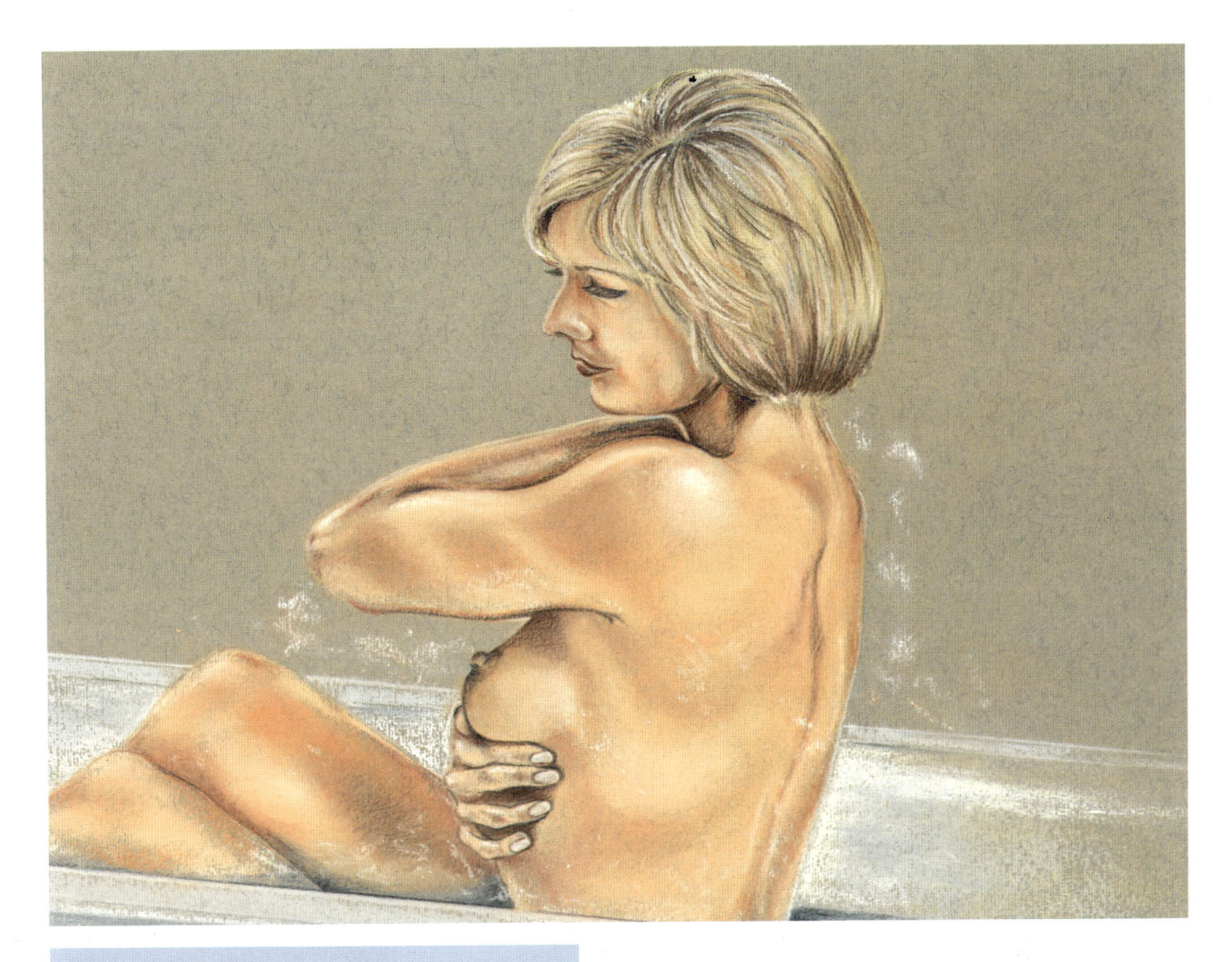

In at the deep end

If you want to give some of the more athletic sexual positions a try, one good way of starting out is to do them in water. Getting in the swim gives you natural buoyancy and prevents you from falling flat on your face. You can try the sitting or kneeling positions in your own bath, if it's large enough, but you'll need a quiet, secluded pool or seaside bay to experiment with standing positions. Water does tend to wash away your natural, necessary body fluids, so take it gently at first. Once you get going, however, lubrication should be no problem.

MANY CULTURES FIND BATHING A HIGHLY SENSUAL EXPERIENCE. SEX IN THE BATH CAN BE GOOD, CLEAN FUN, SO DON'T JUST FANTASIZE ABOUT IT – GIVE IT A GO.

MOVING ON

We've looked at sexual customs around the world, and at sexual practices and sexual positions. But sex is not only a matter of how you do it, to whom and where. Getting it on successfully also depends on how you feel about your own body, what you believe looks attractive and what you think someone else finds exciting and arousing. And when you're not certain that what you've got is enough, what do you use to add a little extra spice to the proceedings? The next chapter looks at all of these areas.

Sex Aids

Do you think you've got what it takes to please your partner in bed? Men the world over seem to share an obsession with the size of their penis, in spite of the fact that women, in surveys and studies in many cultures, say that size is not the main factor for them in sexual satisfaction. So, what can you do if you don't think you measure up?

The human body can be turned on by all kinds of things. Although many of us don't think far beyond vibrators, there's now a huge range of exciting products available

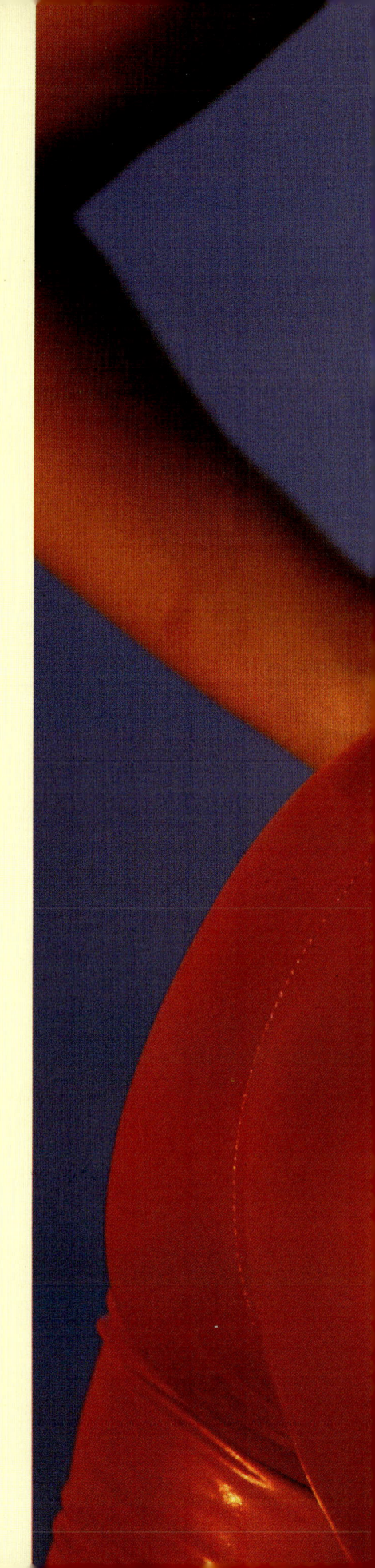

SEX AIDS

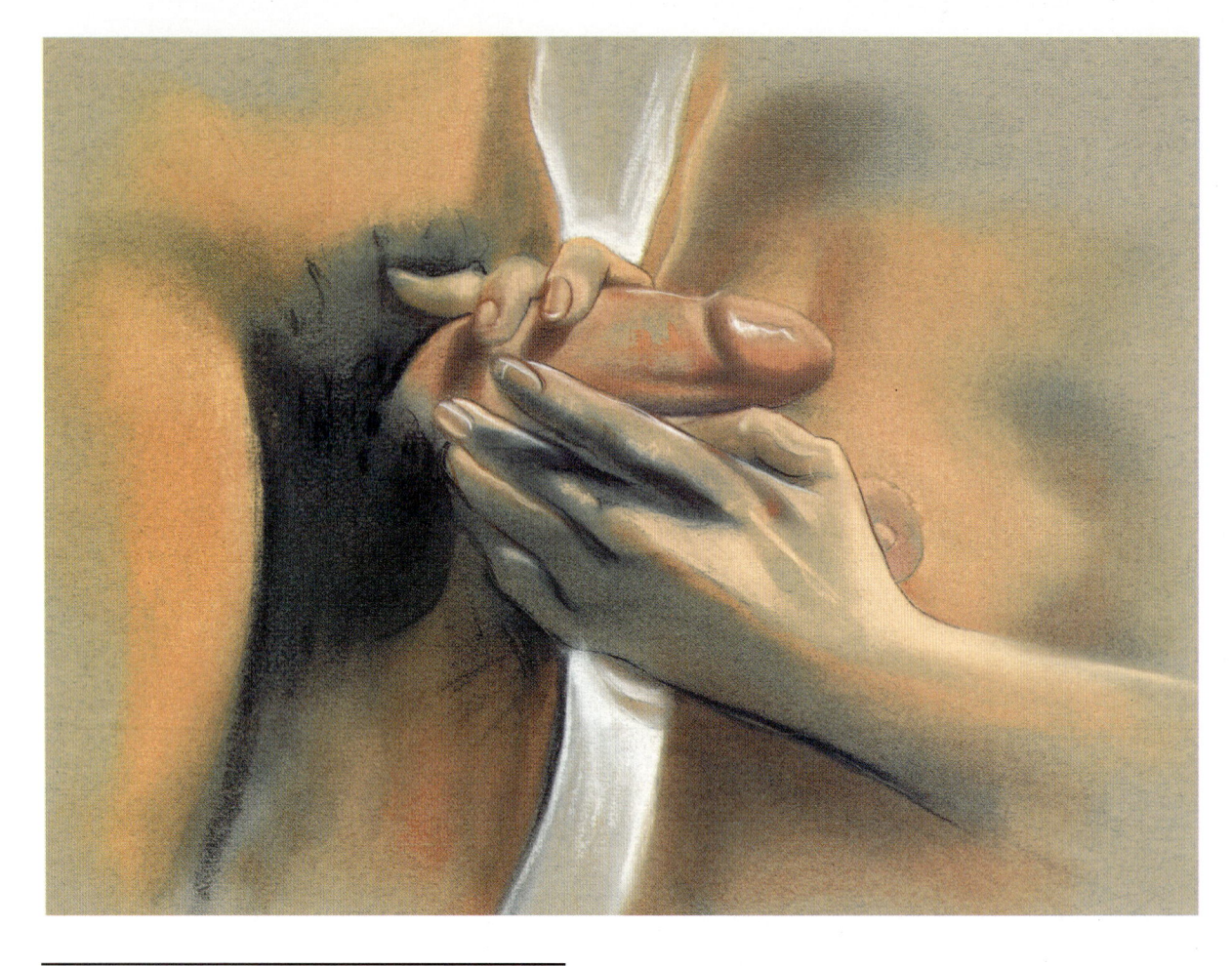

Penis power

A belief that Big is Best is by no means confined to cultures in the West. While Western men and women wear body-hugging clothes to show off their assets, societies such as the Tupinamba in South America and groups in Papua New Guinea wear penis sheaths to show what they've got. The Tupinamba have an interesting cure for any man who thinks he isn't big enough. Macho men of the Tupinamba make poisonous animals bite their penes to make them swell up.

Even if you've got no worries about your manly performance, have you ever wondered if a surgeon could help you to be better endowed? A normal penis is anything between 7 to 11 cm (or 2¾ to 4¼ inches) when flaccid and 14 to 18 cm (5½ to 7¼ inches) when erect. Whatever the measurements, most will end up around the same

THERE ISN'T REALLY A SATISFACTORY METHOD OF MAKING THE PENIS BIGGER, BUT IS SIZE MORE IMPORTANT THAN QUALITY?

rigid size, but many men continue to worry about their penes and some surgeons, particularly in North America, now offer two procedures intended to enhance your assets. In one, part of the structure that anchors the penis to the stomach wall is loosened so that the shaft of the penis extends farther out of the body. Enthusiasts say this can make the penis from one to two centimetres longer. In another procedure, fat can be taken from a man's body and injected into the walls of the penis, making it thicker. In both cases, there are satisfied customers, but it is worth remembering that cosmetic surgery has many drawbacks and dangers.

If you don't want to go under the knife, or allow something with fangs to chow down on your tenderest parts, then what other options are available to you? The *Kama Sutra* suggests bathing the penis with a mixture of plant extracts, aubergine slices and buffalo butter, or with oil boiled with pomegranate seeds, cucumber, aubergines and juices, to make the male member swell. All kinds of suggestions have been made for substances that can be rubbed onto the penis, ranging from tepid water to a mixture of leeches dissolved in oil. Of course, anything that requires you to rub the penis will cause it to swell. However, the result will not last. Your hopes are likely to be the only things enlarged.

In the Western world, hormones are often suggested as a way of increasing the size of a man's penis and testicles. This is on the dubious premise that, since hormonal changes during puberty trigger the growth surge that leads to development, additional hormones later on will make you even bigger. Unfortunately, this is neither a safe nor a correct idea. Hormones are only likely to work if you have had a deficiency, and are only safe if given at the right time, under strict medical supervision.

Adding to your assets

Men who want a temporary increase in size can use a special, padded condom. Some of these also have extensions – a solid tip in the end of the condom that can add some three centimetres to the man's length. These can just be for show, to produce a manly bulge in the trousers, or to lengthen your "reach".

Penis power

Men all over the world are proud of their penes – or not, as the case may be. There have always been plenty of suggestions for ways in which men can increase what they've got, and you can see some of these below. However, few seem to work, and may simply be prolonging a hopeless desire that would be better channelled into making the best, most sensitive use of what Nature has blessed them with.

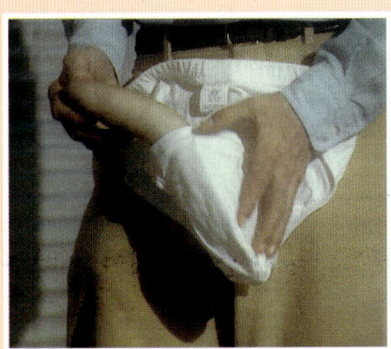

1) UNDERPANTS FITTED WITH A DILDO, OR WITH A FALSE PENIS MADE OF NYLON AND FOAM, MAY GIVE HIM THE OUTLINE HE LONGS FOR

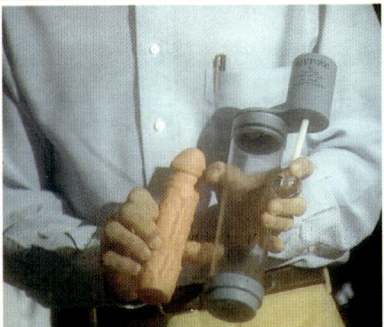

2) PENIS PUMPS CREATE A VACUUM THAT ENCOURAGES THE PENIS TO FILL WITH BLOOD AND ENGORGE – A RATHER TEMPORARY SOLUTION

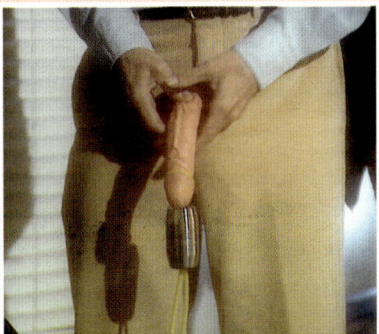

3) SUSPENDING A WEIGHT FROM THE PENIS IS THOUGHT TO LENGTHEN IT BY STRETCHING THE LIGAMENT THAT ATTACHES IT TO THE BELLY

If the man is having difficulty in getting or maintaining an erection long enough to have an orgasm or satisfy his partner, he can also use a penile corset. These are lace-up, open-ended coverings for the penis, made of leather or rubber. They can be used to maintain a wobbly erection – firmer, at least, than it would be without this aid – although the glans might not be as hard and smooth as it would be with full arousal.

> ## Professional guidance
>
> *If you are having erection difficulties, see a doctor before relying on an aid. Aids can be a great help if nothing can be done about the fact that you stay soft, but you might be ignoring an easily dealt with problem that could be important and get worse. Also, remember that a stiff penis isn't always necessary for loving, exciting sex. If penetration of the vagina by the penis isn't possible, consider the joys of non-penetrative sex.*

Another so-called aid to male size is the male developer. These are glass or plastic cylinders with a plastic or rubber tube and bulb attached. According to the claims, they help men increase the size of the penis and are what you will probably receive if you reply to any of the "Watch your penis grow!" advertisements in papers or magazines. You slip the cylinder over the penis and press it tight against the body. You then use the bulb and tube to pump air out of the cylinder, causing a partial vacuum, and an erection. There is also a battery-driven variation where the cylinder moves up and down. Many men use this as a masturbation device, or to start an erection before moving on to loveplay with a partner.

However, "developers" tend to promise far more than they can deliver. They offer false hope to men who are convinced that their world would change for the better if they could add an extra inch to what Nature has provided. No amount of pumping or expanding will cause the penis to enlarge for good because it is made of spongy tissue that enlarges by filling with blood. The "Watch your penis grow" slogan is very clever because you can, indeed, watch it grow – but only from its normally limp state to its normally erect state. When you stop, nothing will have changed permanently.

FEMALE COMPETITION

There are similar "firm 'em up, stick 'em out" developers for women – cone-shaped devices that fit over a breast. Some work by pumping out air, producing a partial vacuum. Others can be fitted to a tap and spray water over the breast. Another style is lined with knobbly bits and is battery-driven. All are supposed to firm up and enlarge the breast. Breasts can expand by as much as a quarter because they are made up of tissue that will flood with blood, and thus swell, during sexual arousal. Any stimulation, whether direct or indirect, will produce the same effect. The manufacturers use this fact to give apparent truth to their amazing claims. But, as with the penis "developer", the breasts return to resting size once you stop using the device. A breast toner can be effective as a masturbatory sex toy – but don't expect anything more.

PUMPING UP

While you can build up and firm up arms, legs, tums and bums, and men can develop their pecs, there are certain parts of the body that can't be altered by exercise. A woman's breasts and a man's penis do not contain muscle tissue, and no amount of pumping iron is going to alter them. Breasts may even decrease in size after exercise, because they contain pads of fat, which can burn off just like fat on any other part of the body. However, as

WESTERN CULTURE IS OBSESSED WITH LARGE BREASTS, BUT BEAUTY SHOULD BE A MATTER OF PERSONAL TASTE

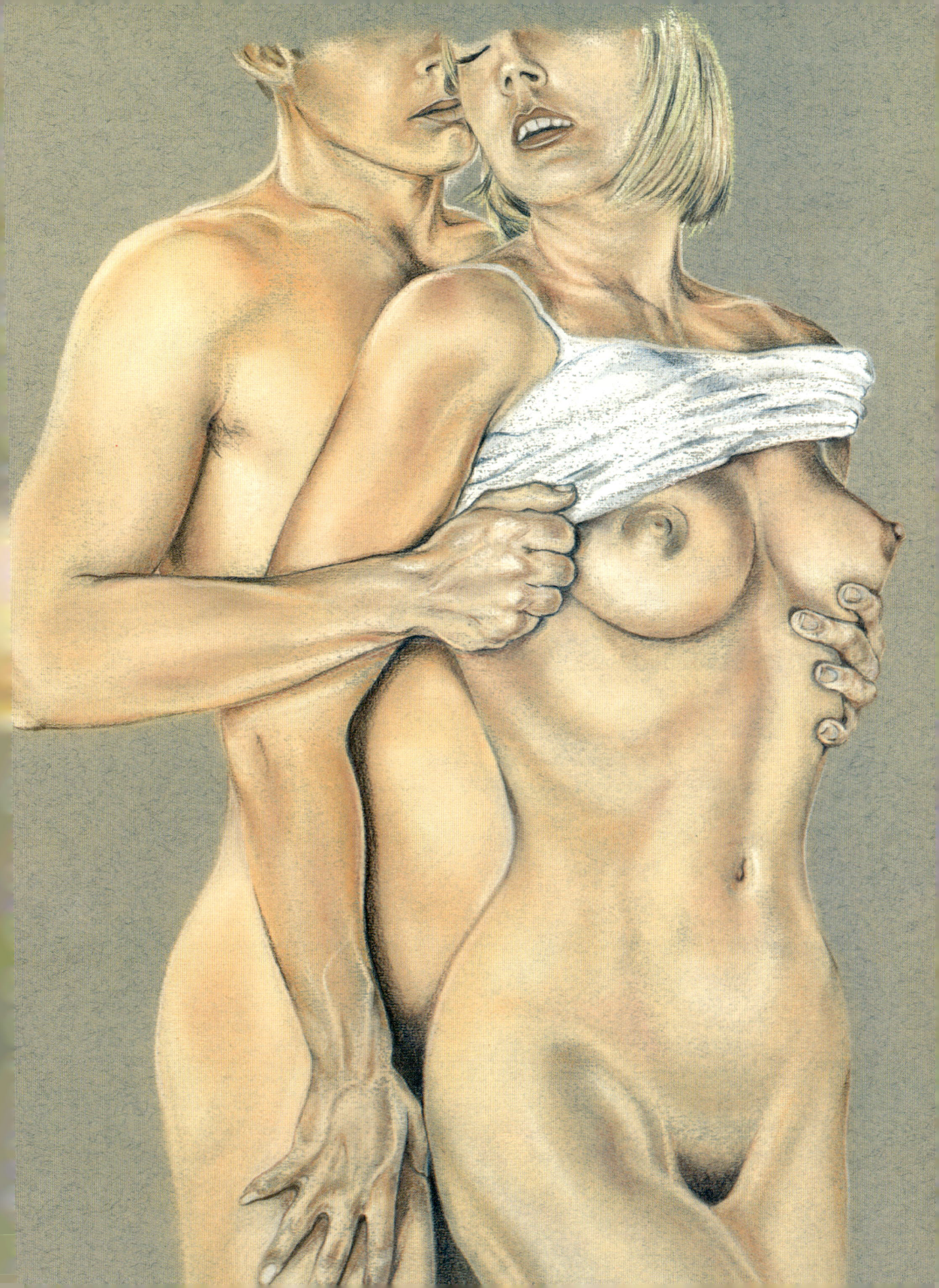

Sexual muscle-flexing

You can do these exercises at any time and in any position, with very little obvious effort. All you need to do is to pull up the muscle as if you were trying to stop a flow of urine. You can best practise this exercise by doing just that. Go to the toilet and, as you start to pass water, stop and start the stream. You don't have to clench your fists or buttocks, curl your toes or make faces to be doing this movement strongly enough. Just stop and start, and once you have the sensations identified, try the exercise as you go about your daily routine – squeeze and release, squeeze and release. Do it 15 to 20 times each hour.

After a few months of regular flexing, you will notice a difference. And so will your partner, particularly if you continue doing your exercises while making love. A woman can't possibly tighten hard enough to hurt her man, but she certainly can tighten enough for him to feel it deliciously. Try it, timing your movements to his orgasm. A man can use the control to lengthen the time he can make love before he comes.

you read in Chapter 1, you would be able to firm up the pectoral muscles that lie underneath the breasts, giving the breasts a firmer platform from which to hang. Exercise may also give you better posture and so allow you to thrust out what you do have to better effect.

PELVIC MUSCLE EXERCISES

There is one muscle women and men can develop that *can* have a specific effect on your love-life. The pubococcygeus muscle is a broad band of tissue that sweeps from the pelvic bone to the tailbone or coccyx. In women, it supports the pelvic organs, and if it becomes slack, you can become unable to hold your water. You may then dribble a few drops whenever you laugh, cough, sneeze or jump. Your vagina may also feel slack, so that both you and your partner may find sex less satisfying. Ultimately, the bladder or the womb may slump downwards into the vagina in a prolapse.

One gynaecologist, Arnold Kegel, suggested that women could avoid these problems by doing a set of exercises now called Kegel exercises. You can buy a Kegel exerciser – sometimes described as a "barbell" for the vagina – although it isn't really necessary to have one to do this exercise successfully. By putting something in the vagina however, you would have something to squeeze against, and you could use a vibrator, a dildo or love eggs (see later in the chapter) for this purpose.

Men are reputed to have an even more dramatic sexual reaction to developing their pubococcygeus muscle. During lovemaking, if the man has control over this muscle, he can then practise Tantric sex, where ejaculation is held off or prevented, but the man can still have several orgasms, one after the other. Practitioners of Tantric sex say that learning to control this muscle can improve sexual powers to an awesome degree.

UNDER THE KNIFE

In recent years, certainly in the West, it has become increasingly trendy to have your less attractive physical features restructured by the plastic surgeons. You may not want to go as far as some celebrities of the show business or fashion scenes, but you may feel there is at least one part of your body you'd like to be different – say, a firmer rear, better-shaped breasts or neater genitals. So, what can surgeons do to help you to gild your particular lily and improve your sex-life?

Surgery can help our love-life in two ways. It can improve appearances so that we look better and therefore feel more confident and sexier. Or it can correct a physical problem that otherwise would stop or hinder us having sex at all. Men can have their version of breast enlargement to give themselves muscular looking "pecs", but generally, aside from corrective surgery or a vasectomy, most males go into the operating theatre for either a circumcision or a prosthesis.

Male circumcision

Male circumcision is the surgical removal of the foreskin – the loose skin covering the end of the penis. Circumcision is known to date back to the ancient Egyptians, possibly further, and may be done for religious, hygienic or medical purposes. The two main medical reasons for circumcision are phimosis (difficulty in drawing back the foreskin) and paraphimosis (the inability to return it over the glans once you have drawn it back). It is estimated that over half of all men living today have been circumcised. Circumcision is common among Muslims and Jews, throughout most of the Middle East and Africa – although not in central or East Africa – and in Polynesia.

Cultural differences

Among the Nandi of Kenya, the foreskin is burnt off with a hot coal. Others trim it with a knife, while the Marquesans of the central Pacific slit the foreskin, supposedly to make it easier for men to keep clean. Circumcision is done at different times in different cultures. In traditional Jewish families, it is performed on the eighth day after childbirth. In many Polynesian and African societies, it is performed as a part of the rites of passage, around puberty. Among some groups, a male who hasn't been circumcised isn't considered an adult and no woman will consider having sex with him or marrying him.

The foreskin is not the only part of the male sex organs that may be cut. In Ethiopia, the Janjero remove one testicle in the belief that men with two will father twins, who are considered bad luck. The Mangaians and some other Polynesian societies make a cut the entire length of the penis. When the wound is healed, a cord is tied round the end of the foreskin and the knot is only loosened for passing water and making love. Again, a male who has not had this operation is not considered to have matured from a boy into a man.

Male circumcision is often seen as a direct aid to male sexual pleasure. It's said to make the glans or head of the penis slightly less sensitive, so allowing the man to make love for longer. It's also thought by some to have health benefits for men and their partners. Circumcised men are less likely to suffer cancer of the penis and some sexually transmitted diseases, and their female sexual partners are less at risk of cancer of the cervix. What's still in doubt is whether this is strictly because of the circumcision or has more to do with the better hygiene and less sexual activity that is usually found in traditionally circumcised groups or societies.

However, there are those who oppose circumcision and see it as a mutilating operation. Men who have been circumcised may resent their parents for having had it done to them, seeing it as a castrating and controlling action. They may also claim that the exposed glans becomes slightly less sensitive, and that this spoils lovemaking for them and their partners.

Female circumcision

In many of the cultures that circumcise their men, there is a ritual operation done on female children too, also called circumcision. The modern Western concept of female circumcision is an operation to free the clitoris from any tissue that surrounds and fixes it, or to remove part of the clitoral hood. Some women report greater sensitivity after this and both men and women may say they can find the appearance of an exposed clitoris exciting. However, even though you might like the appearance, you might not be too charmed with the physical sensations the procedure can produce. Unlike the penis, the clitoris shrinks and retreats inside its protective fold of skin as orgasm approaches, and most women would find that a naked clitoris would become so tender at that point in intercourse that any direct touch would be painful rather than pleasant.

Another modern operation sometimes performed on female genitals is labia restructuring, done to reduce and tidy-up the inner and outer fleshy lips on each side of the vagina. This can be a helpful operation for women who suffer discomfort from large labia that hang down too far. However, it is worth noting that, among cultures such as the Tswana from Botswana, the Thonga from Mozambique, the Marquesans and the Trukese, such a physical feature is prized and envied.

Where is it done?

Female circumcision is carried out in the Sudan, United Arab Emirates, Oman, Bahrain, South Yemen, Somalia, Djibouti, Southern Egypt, Eritrea/Ethiopia, Mali and across central Africa.

True female circumcision is another procedure entirely and a better name for it is genital mutilation. There are several types of female circumcision. One is excision, in which the clitoris and all or part of the labia minora are cut away. Another is infibulation, where the clitoris, the labia minora and part of the labia majora are cut away and the vaginal opening mostly stitched up. The Nandi, who burn off the male foreskin with a hot coal, remove their girls' clitori in the same manner. In countries such as Kenya, female circumcision has been banned by law but since men refuse to marry uncircumcised women, mothers will break the law to have their daughters operated on. In Yorubaland, it's believed that a woman cannot give birth to a live baby if her clitoris is intact. But in the Sudan, new generation men do prefer wives who are uncircumcised or who have had the "sunna" method of circumcision, where only the female foreskin is removed.

As with male circumcision, many explanations are given for the custom, from religion to hygiene. One reason is likely to be to keep women from having sex before marriage and keep them faithful afterwards. Although the network of nerve endings in the female genitals extends beyond the clitoris itself, women who have had this operation would seem to experience far less pleasurable response than women who have not. In addition, the operation leaves scar tissue that is painful. Genital mutilation frequently leads to infections and a lasting legacy of ill health.

Restored "virginity"

In some cultures, a high premium is placed on female virginity. Failure to produce "proof" of this, in the shape of a tight vagina and bleeding on a wedding night, can mean becoming a social outcast. While some cultures tighten a girl's vagina by putting astringents on it, there is also a new operation, called hymenoplasty, which replaces the hymen by using skin grafts. Sexually experienced women can then give a later partner some semblance of virginity and re-enact a traditional bridal night.

Hymenectomy

Hymenectomy is a minor operation that breaks the hymen surgically, in order to make lovemaking possible. The hymen, a fold of membrane that partly blocks off the vagina, is usually thin and flexible. With the physically active lives of today's young women, or from self-exploration or tampon use, it often stretches and breaks long before a girl first has intercourse. But in some girls, the membrane is tough, and first attempts at intercourse are very painful. If the membrane resists gentle attempts to loosen it, it can be separated with hymenectomy.

A bad sign

In many cultures, taking a woman's maidenhead is seen to be so fraught with spiritual significance that any man who first has sex with her could be courting terrible misfortune. So, a girl may have her maidenhead stretched or broken when she is a baby, or as part of her coming of age ritual. It may be done by an old woman, as in some African societies, or by an old and impotent man. In Hindu, Indonesian and Native South American societies, it is done when baby girls are one month old.

MALE AIDS

Men can now have an implant in the penis to create an erection when a physical problem prevents the man from having one under his own steam. There are three main groups of penile prosthesis currently on offer. In one type, two silicone rods are implanted in the penis. The rods are either hinged at the base or contain a flexible metal coil. When an erection is wanted, the man or his partner simply straightens the penis. In the second type, the penis is implanted with two hollow shafts, connected to reservoirs filled with fluid. Any pressure on the tip of the penis causes a pump to flood the shafts, making the penis stand up. The third group is the inflatables. These have a pair of inflatable silicone cylinders in the shaft of the penis with a pump implanted in the scrotum and a reservoir buried behind the abdominal muscle. The three parts are connected by silicone tubing. You get an erection by squeezing the scrotal pump, which then moves fluid from the reservoir into the cylinders in the shaft. The results are a very realistic, firm erection with some increase in length and girth to the penis.

Unfortunately, surgery for any type of prosthesis implant causes irreversible damage. A normal erection won't be possible again, so it's not advisable just because you think what you have to offer doesn't seem firm or big enough to fulfil your sexual fantasies.

BREAST ENLARGEMENT

Of course, women can have their breasts permanently enlarged or firmed up by surgery that inserts silicone or polyurethane bags containing silicone gel or saline water. The bags are placed either between the existing breast tissue and the muscle that lies against the ribs, or between muscle and ribs. The implant pushes out the woman's natural breast tissue to create the desired fuller shape. Implants don't stop a woman being able to breastfeed, and they don't increase the risk of breast cancer or mask other symptoms such as breast lumps. The majority of implants don't affect feeling in the breast either, although some 10% of women report a temporary or permanent loss of feeling in the nipples. A further undesirable effect can be a build-up of scar tissue around the implant, making the breasts hard and unnaturally regular in appearance.

BREAST REDUCTION

In spite of all the stale male jokes, some women feel they have been over-endowed and can suffer discomfort from having very large breasts. The surgical solution is an operation to remove tissue from the breasts, making them smaller and firmer. An incision is made in the lower half of the breast and excess tissue is cut away. The nipple and the surrounding area is moved upwards, and the whole is sewn back together. The operation might stop any embarrassment, pain or tenderness for a woman, but the down side is that it also stops any chance of future breastfeeding and, in most cases, the nipples will be less sensitive.

NIPPLES

Nipples are another area where many women feel they fall short of the ideal. Nipples are not really meant to stand out except when stimulated, but many women, or their men, feel something is wrong if they do not match up to the organ stop variety shown in erotic pictures. The surgery to correct inverted nipples and to make them stand out involves cutting through the areola (the dark area around the nipple) and separating the shortened milk ducts that pull the nipple flat against the surface or inside the breast. This procedure always prevents breastfeeding in the future and will certainly reduce sensation or even destroy it altogether.

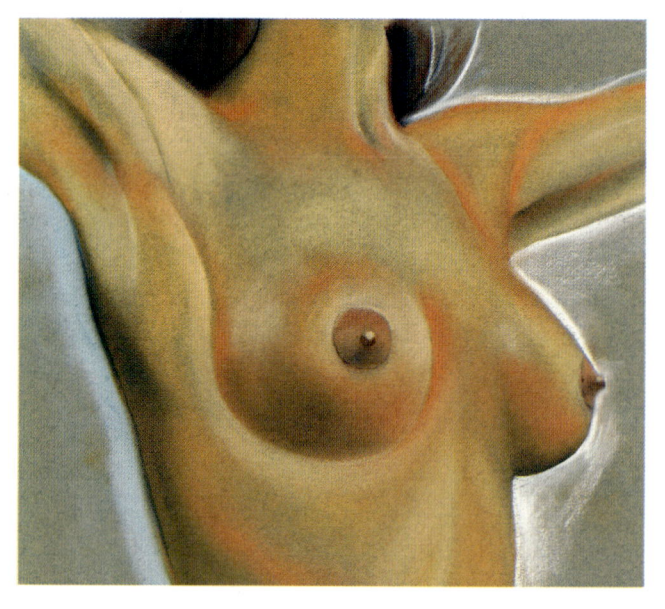

THE APPEARANCE AND TEXTURE OF THE FEMALE BREAST VARIES ENORMOUSLY, AS DO THE THINGS THAT MAKE PEOPLE FEEL COMFORTABLE AND GOOD ABOUT THEMSELVES. IN THE WEST TODAY, JUST AS MANY WOMEN ARE ASKING FOR BREAST REDUCTION OPERATIONS AS FOR BREAST ENLARGEMENT

Think about it first

Having bits tightened up, moved around or taken off will not guarantee your becoming a social lion or a sexual gold medalist. A doctor does not always have to have specialist qualifications to practise cosmetic surgery, and there are practitioners galore who are far more interested in your bank account than in your physical or emotional well-being. The only safe way to approach cosmetic surgery is to get yourself referred to a reputable surgeon through your regular general practitioner. And you should only take this step after you have had counselling or given considerable thought to whether this action is the right one for you.

IN THE MOOD

Tradition tells of a bewildering array of foods and substances you can eat or drink that are supposed to get you going. The Koreans and Chinese believe ginseng does the trick, the Inuit of Greenland use the bill knob of the king eider, Hindus recommend lotus flower pollen, Arabs speak highly of cinnamon and Europeans cry the virtues of caviar, celery, lavender, licorice – and chocolate, if confectionery sales around Valentine's Day are anything to go by! Asparagus, bananas, and rhinoceros horn are claimed to help the man hold up his end; oysters, figs and marrow bone jelly are suggested as being helpful to women. At some time or other, all over the world, just about any plant or substance has been believed to be aphrodisiac.

Aphrodisiacs are supposed to work by encouraging an erection in the man or lubrication in the woman, and sensations of heat and urgency in both. Many cultures recommend "hot" foods – for example, a type of wild ginger found in the

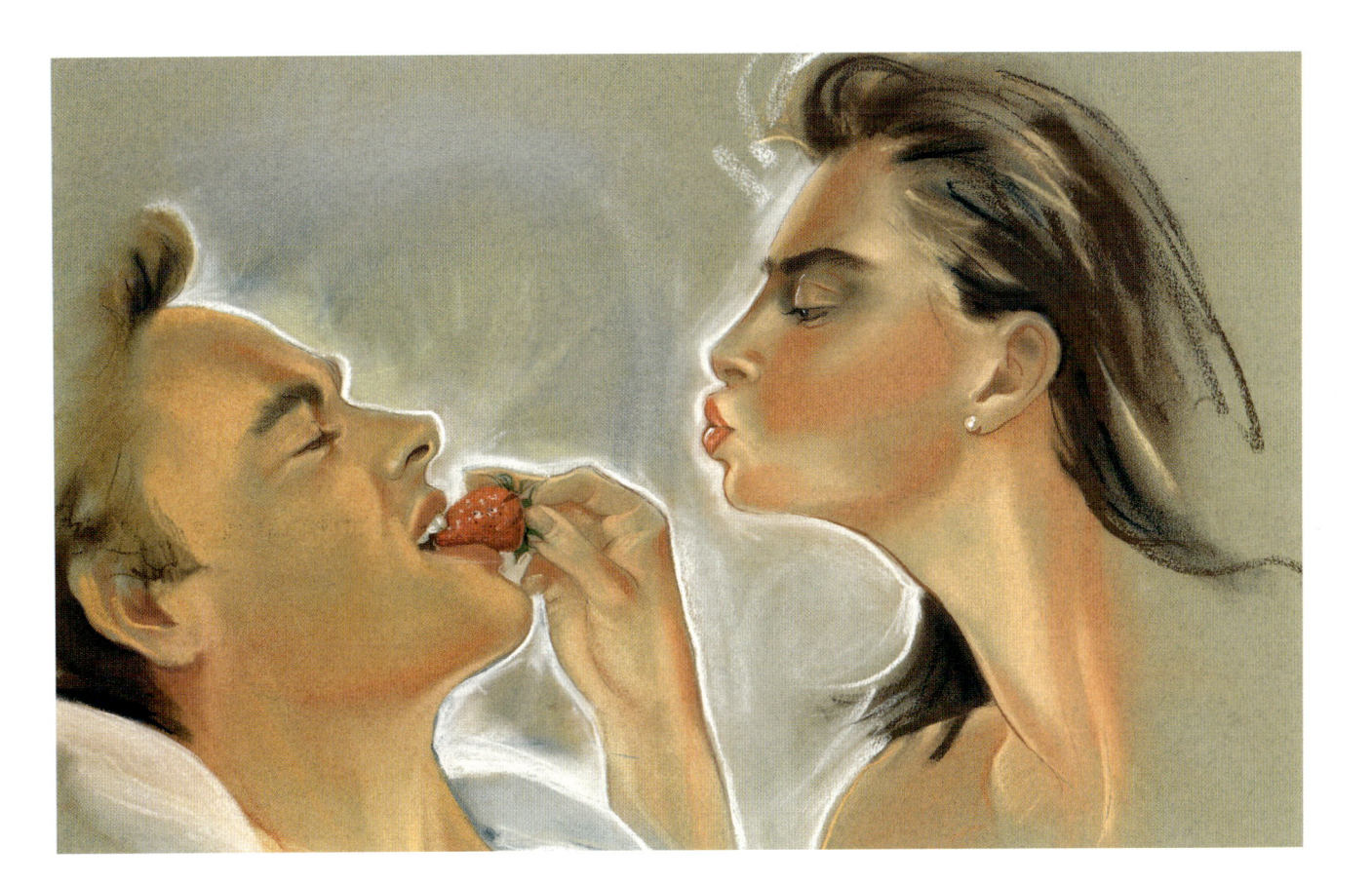

Solomon Islands is believed to be particularly effective by the locals. Or indulgent and enjoyable tastes such as spices and herbs, sweetmeats, honey and sugar. Other foods might be thought to work by "sympathetic magic" – rhino horn, asparagus, bananas and ginseng are all phallic in shape. Oysters, figs and marrow bones have the smell or the appearance of a woman's vulva or vagina when she is aroused and ready for love.

Do they work? Any substance that peps us up can act as an aphrodisiac in helping us to feel livelier and sexier. There are substances that can be swallowed or rubbed on the skin that may give a feeling of tingling or warmth to the genitals and be thought to be aphrodisiac. However, slipping your partner one of these foods is unlikely to do the trick unless you pointed out what it was supposed to do! Your best bet would be to light the candles, serve a meal of caviar, asparagus spears and quails' eggs, and make sure

THE SENSITIVITY OF OUR LIPS AND TASTE BUDS IS SUCH THAT SHARING FOOD CAN BE AS EXCITING AS, AND A GOOD PRELUDE TO, ACTUALLY MAKING LOVE

there's a large box of chocolate truffles on the bedroom table. It may work, but whether from chemical reaction or expectation... who knows? (And if it does work, who cares?)

Eating in bed

Plenty of fish, fresh fruit and vegetables would have a genuine effect on your well-being and so could improve your sexual interest and abilities. But it has to be admitted that sharing a nut cutlet and a calorie-counted salad can't match the suggestive powers of slurping a dozen oysters together before climbing between the sheets. The general rule seems to be that if you don't need them, they could be fun. If you do need them, they probably won't work.

SEX AIDS

SPRAY-ON SEX

Two Australian doctors appear to have accidentally discovered an extremely unlikely, but effective, aphrodisiac. A female patient was given a nasal spray containing oxytocin, the hormone produced by the body to stimulate milk production. Two hours after using the spray she reported that she was overcome with intense sexual desire. However, when she used the spray on another occasion, it had no such startling effect. The patient had stopped taking the contraceptive Pill in the interval and this may explain the difference in her reactions.

SPANISH FLY

Spanish Fly is often suggested as a sex aid. The active ingredient is cantharidin, a substance made from powdered, dried beetles. Spanish Fly might be offered as a powder to add to food or drink, as a ready-mixed solution with alcohol or as a tablet. When swallowed, it's supposed to heat up your sexual organs, making you insatiable. Cantharidin does have a warming effect, but only by inflaming and damaging the bladder and water passage. Men have died as a result of using Spanish Fly and many people have been temporarily or permanently damaged by it. It's extremely dangerous.

Oil you need is love

Try this for a night of passion. Buy yourself a ready-mixed bottle of aromatherapy oil, or mix your own from a bottle of "carrier" oil such as almond, vegetable or sunflower oil and an essential oil. The usual mix is 3 parts essential oil to 100 parts carrier oil. The essential oils distilled from black pepper, cardamom, jasmine, juniper, orange blossom, patchouli, clary sage, rose, sandalwood and ylang-ylang are all reputed to be aphrodisiac. Put a towel down on the bed, or on the floor, pour a handful onto your mate and get stroking. When your lover is good and slippery, and well relaxed, change places. Experiment so that you can both discover just what feels good and what feels even better. And if all that kneading, stroking and sliding about leads to more intimate pleasures... well, what a surprise!

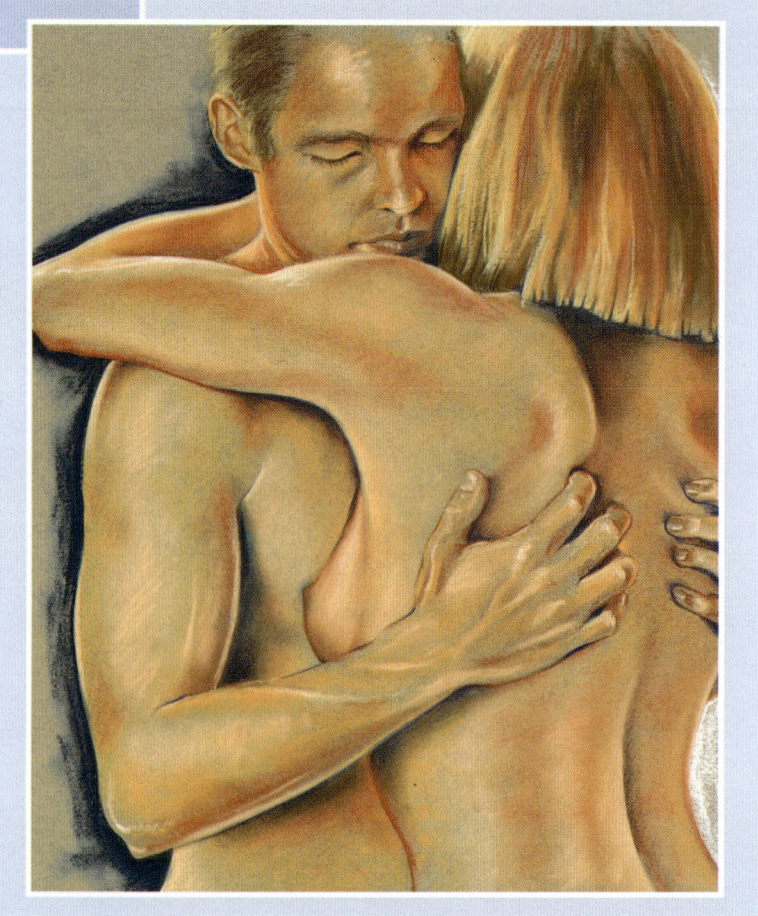

THE SLIPPERY SENSATIONS AND AROUSING SCENTS OF AROMATHERAPY OILS CAN DO MUCH TO PUT YOU IN THE MOOD FOR LOVE

Aromatherapy

Substances don't have to be swallowed to have aphrodisiac properties, according to Eastern practitioners. Aromatherapy enthusiasts say that essential oils distilled from flowers, trees, herbs and fruits can have an effect, whether they are absorbed into the body through the skin, during massage or bathing, or as perfume and incense. They can be heated on a special burner or on rings that rest on a light bulb, releasing the fragrance. Different oils are said to have different effects and some are claimed to be aphrodisiac.

Getting under your skin?

There can be no doubt that the largest of our organs – our skin – is not as waterproof as we might think. Substances put on the skin can seep through into the bloodstream, depending on what they contain and how long they stay in contact with the surface. Conventional medicine now makes use of this in delivering Hormone Replacement Therapy (HRT), and some drugs for heart disease, through patches stuck in place on the chest or bottom to allow a steady, measured amount to be absorbed. A substance absorbed in this way travels directly into the bloodstream without having to go through the stomach and liver. This means that a small amount can go a long way and have a quick effect.

Tattoos

In both Eastern and Western societies, men and women decorate their skin as a way of signalling sexual attraction. In societies such as Oceania or in Zaire, this takes the form of elaborate scars, tattoos or painted designs. Non-Western societies often tattoo young people as part of the coming of age ritual. No anaesthetic is used, in order to test how well someone can stand up to pain.

You can have a tattoo any place where you have skin. Tattoos intended as sexual adornment are often found on buttocks, breasts and on the lower belly. Genital tattoos – on the penis or the pubic mound – are found in some Oceanic cultures and are mainly done on women, and this is also true of the Mongo in Africa. One king of Tonga, however, was said to have tattoos all over the head of his penis, as proof of his ability to ignore pain. Romeos in Mangaia will have a picture of a vulva tattooed on their penes, to boast about their swordsmanship. In the West, many people take a delight in having a tattoo in a place that only their partner will see.

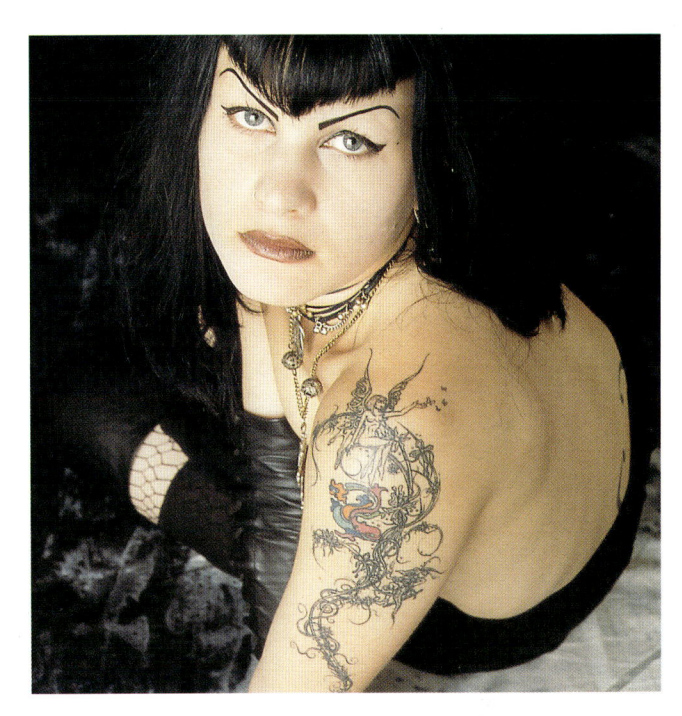

IN SOME SOCIETIES, SKIN DESIGNS RELATE TO SOCIAL STATUS. THEY ARE INCREASINGLY FASHIONABLE IN THE WEST

Picture this...

Try painting a small design, somewhere only your lover will see it – on your penis, around a nipple, on your backside. Use washable inks, make-up or a removable, stick-on tattoo. If you both like the effect, you could always consider making it permanent!

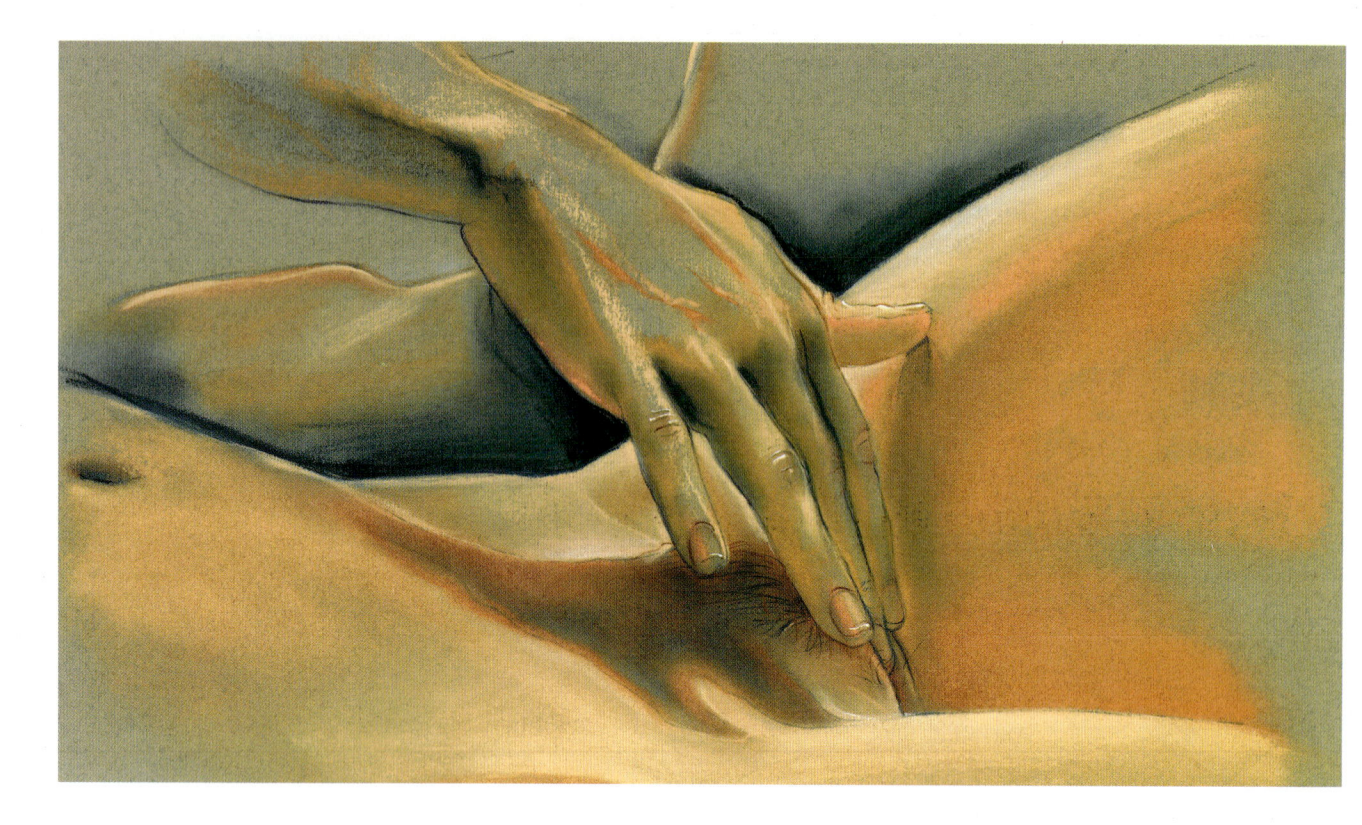

Try something new with your body hair – cutting it, growing it, or going totally bare!

BODY HAIRDRESSING

A less permanent way of beautifying the genitals is cutting, shaving or cultivating the pubic hair. Hair is very sexy, and the length of your hair and how you wear it can send powerful sexual signals to other people. Body hair is often even more important than head hair. Human beings may have body hair as a form of insulation – left over from our animal ancestry. The patches that are left have a second function in that they often act as traps for pheromones. These are chemicals present in sweat that attract the opposite sex. They are particularly rich in the sweat under the arms and around the genitals. In some cultures, women's underarm hair and hair on the legs, far from being thought unfeminine, is seen as raunchy and sexy. In various other societies, pubic hair is removed as a way of focusing attention on the genitals.

A change of style

See if you and your partner fancy a change in the way you manage your body hair. You could go halfway to start. Using nail scissors, gently clip your pubic hair short and see if you like the effect. Or try shaving the top of the pubic hair to produce a shape – a heart, perhaps, or the apex of a diamond. If you do decide on shaving, use a sharp razor, plenty of soap, and go slowly and gently. The best technique is to clip the hair short first, and then shave the remaining stubble. You could use depilatory cream (do a patch-test first on nearby skin) for outer areas, but do not allow it to come into contact with the internal mucous membranes. Be especially careful shaving the scrotum. Because this area is wrinkled, it is difficult to shave without cutting yourself. Four hands – to stretch, soap and hold bits out of the way – are better than two!

SEX TOYS

In general, the more sexually reticent cultures, such as the British and the North Americans, seem to feel that all you need for a good sex life are a man, a woman, an erection and a bed. Other societies suggest that to play the game of love to its full, a few more toys increase the fun.

Sex toys are an accepted part of the arts of love around the world. The Tikopia of the Pacific and the Zande from Sudan encourage the use of bananas and roots as dildos or penis substitutes. These are used by women to learn their sexual responses and to please themselves, but also as a part of loving between a couple. Dildos are hardly new. They are shown in ancient Babylonian sculpture, on Greek pottery and mentioned in the Bible. Dildos are now usually made out of plastic or latex, but around the world they may come in ivory, wood or glass. In one early Japanese erotic manual you can find instructions on making your own – from a carrot.

Modern high-tech can transform the humble dildo into a supercharged, battery- or mains-driven sex machine – the vibrator. These come in several basic forms. There are penis-shaped vibrators, which can be anything from 13 cm long and 2-3 cm in diameter to an enormous 31 cm with a proportionately massive girth. Some are smooth and made of hard plastic or with a metallic

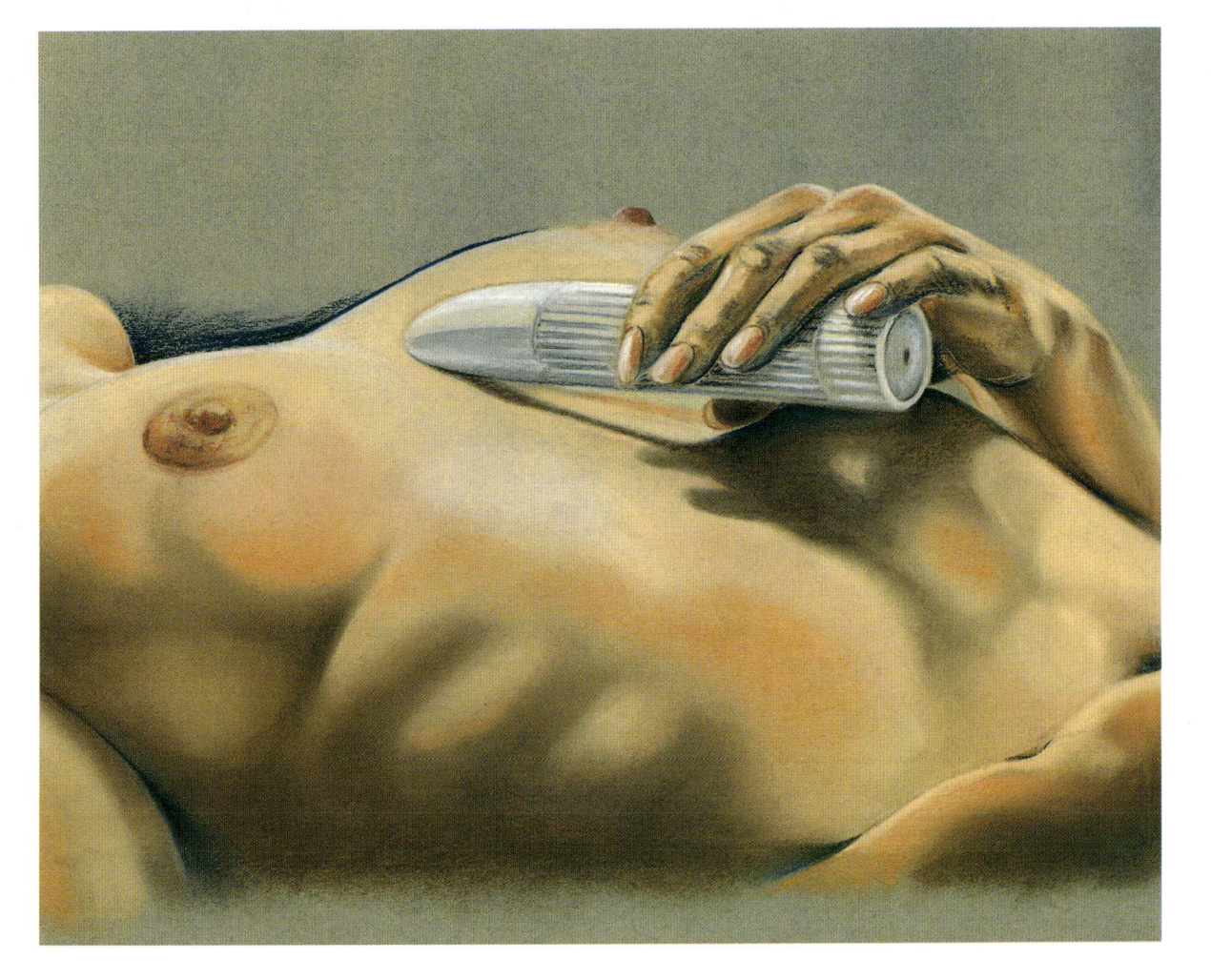

PENIS-SHAPED VIBRATORS ARE NOT ONLY FOR VAGINAL USE. THEY CAN BE USED IN AS MANY WAYS AS THERE ARE PLACES WHERE YOU AND YOUR PARTNER LIKE BEING TOUCHED

finish. Some have grooves, ribbing or knobbly bumps. Others are veined to look like a penis and are made of soft latex to give a flesh-like texture. You can also get soft latex or rubber covers to transform a hard, smooth vibrator into a soft, veined one. Some penis-shaped vibrators come with an extra bit on the base that is designed to rub against the clitoris; others contain beads beneath a soft outer skin, or have rings of beads set in the shaft. A further variation has a distinct bend at the end, supposedly to touch the G-spot, and another has a second prong to enter the back passage at the same time as the main part enters the vagina. Penis-shaped vibrators can move side-to-side, up-and-down, or rotate, or a combination of these. Some will heat up, some have a reservoir that can be filled with warm liquid to be squirted out like an ejaculation, and some will even glow in the dark.

Not all vibrators are made to resemble the penis. The "butterfly" is an oblong pad with straps, shaped to fit snugly over the clitoris and vagina. Another model is shaped like a small egg and is connected by a cord to a separate battery pack.

All these vibrators are supposedly designed with women in mind and for use in the vagina or on and around the clitoris. But vibrators are made with the male anatomy in mind, too. For example, there is a ring that clips around the penis, holding a small vibrating lozenge against the base of the shaft. Others are designed as artificial vaginas. These are latex or rubber tubes, smooth on the inside or lined with soft projections. Some can "pump up" to increase pressure around the penis; some are shaped like a woman's head to give the user the impression of having oral sex.

LOVE EGGS

Love eggs are believed to have been invented by the Japanese. They consist of two hollow balls joined by a cord, and may contain smaller balls or weights that move round inside the smooth shells. Put into the vagina, love eggs are supposed to bring you to a climax, or to keep you in a state of constant sexual arousal. Having something just inside the vagina is likely to give you interesting sensations. An object pressing wide the normally collapsed tube of the vagina could cause the clitoris to move against its protective hood – or indeed, press it up against clothing.

THAI BEADS

Thai beads are made up of several plastic beads, either on a string or a flexible rod. You place them in the back passage and gently move them in and out or vibrate them during sexual arousal. They can also be slowly, or quickly, pulled out as you climax. The anus and rectum are sensitive, and having something resting in and rubbing against the sides of this opening can be pleasant. Research has shown that contractions at orgasm squeeze the rectum shut in both men and women, so putting something into this passage can obviously add to the excitement for many people.

A BIT OF SLAP AND TICKLE

Ticklers and clitoral stimulators are used the world over to give women extra sensation during lovemaking. Many women find that the normal action of intercourse, with the penis thrusting in and out of the vagina, doesn't actually hit the right spot. Direct touching or rubbing of the clitoris itself may be preferred. So too may increased sensation in the vagina. This can be done by either partner using their fingers, or by using a clitoral stimulator or a "French tickler".

Ticklers are made of metal, animal skin or, in the Western world, plastic or rubber. They consist either of a ring to slide up the shaft of the penis, to be worn behind the glans or at the base of the shaft, or a covering for the entire shaft. The device's surface texture provides vaginal stimulation, brushes against the entrance to the vagina as the man pushes in or out, or rubs against the clitoris itself.

Switch on, turn on

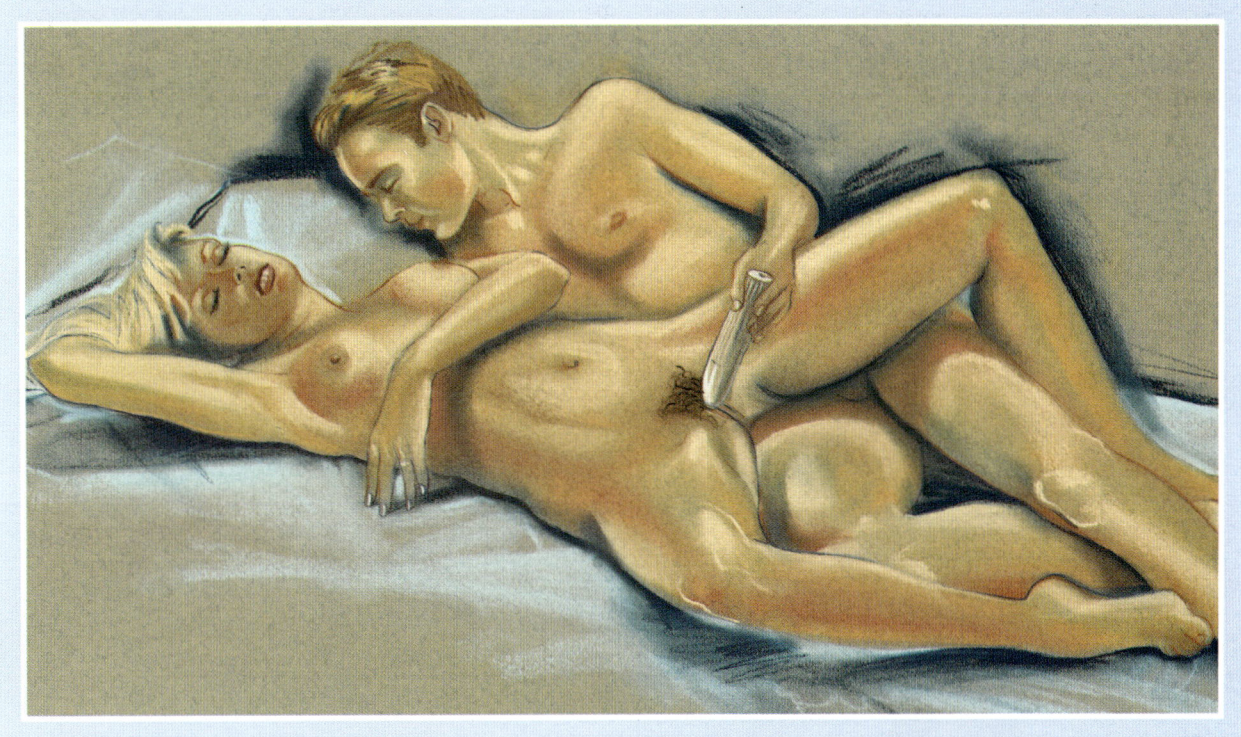

TRY OUT A VIBRATOR WITH YOUR PARTNER AND TELL EACH OTHER WHAT YOU LIKE BEST

Make sure you are warm and comfortable, and if your vibrator has several speeds, start with the slowest. Pass the vibrator gently over your body, avoiding the obvious spots such as nipples and genitals. Try that again, pressing harder. Increase the speed and go again.

If your partner is with you, give them the vibrator and let them try the same self-exploration. Then have your partner repeat the exercise on you and see if having someone else doing it makes it feel different. Experiment and tell each other which touches are pleasurable, and which are exciting. Don't worry if you find that the sensations or the situation makes you giggle.

Now move on to the more obvious places. Try pressing the vibrator against nipples, on ear lobes and lips, on the inside of the legs and around the back passage entrance or the lower back. Women are likely to find it arousing to have the vibrator tip passed over the labia and around the clitoris. Men are likely to find it exciting to have the length of the vibrator pressed against the shaft of the penis, or the tip passed around or pressed against the glans. They may also find it stimulating to have the tip pressed against the scrotum and against the skin immediately behind it.

Some vibrators are clearly labelled as being waterproof and can be used with soap and water. If you have one of these, make your explorations in the bath (you must *make sure that it is labelled as waterproof first*). The warmth and slipperiness of bathtime can greatly increase your pleasure.

BODY PIERCING

In many parts of the world, especially Indonesia and the South Pacific, they make a permanent addition to the penis to create a type of tickler. The practice of inserting bits of bamboo, stones, pearls or metal balls into cuts made along the shaft of the penis or under the glans is common. In the Philippines and Borneo, bars are inserted through the penis to secure metal rings. Genital jewellery isn't only about sensation, however. It may also serve to attract and beautify. Trukese women insert bells into their labia, and in Burma men put tiny bronze bells in their penes, which tinkle and ring as they walk – is this the origin of the catchphrase "Ring my bell!"?

We are all familiar with the sight of pierced ears. This type of piercing allows you to wear earrings as an attractive adornment, but many people find the fact of piercing rather sexy in itself. And others report that you can use the presence of jewellery to create pleasurable sensations. Gently tweaking at sensitive earlobes can be very stimulating. So why stop at ears? Cultures all over the world have pierced nipples and other parts of the body for centuries. Both men and women pierce ears, lower lips, noses and cheeks, but it is also possible to pierce nipples, navels and the sexual organs. Women can be pierced through both the inner and the outer labia, through the clitoris hood or through the clitoris itself.

An ancient practice

The Kama Sutra *says that "people of the Southern countries think that true sexual pleasure cannot be obtained without piercing the penis, and they therefore cause it to be pierced like the lobes of the ears." The practice continues today.*

Penis piercings are quite common in Europe, America and Japan, not only for decoration but also to enhance sensation during sex. This can be done through the foreskin, either in such a way as to pass a ring or barbell through to prevent the foreskin being skinned back or retracted, or so that a ring can be inserted allowing the foreskin to move unimpeded. The frenum – the loose bridge of flesh beneath the glans – can also be pierced. The most popular male genital piercing is the "Prince Albert". In this, a hole is made through the glans into the urethra just above the frenum. A ring is then worn that comes out of the tip of the penis and circles round underneath. Men can also have holes pierced straight through the glans, through the scrotal sac, at the base of the belly, just above the penis, or in the ridge of flesh behind the scrotum that lies in front of the back passage entrance – this last variation originated in the South Pacific.

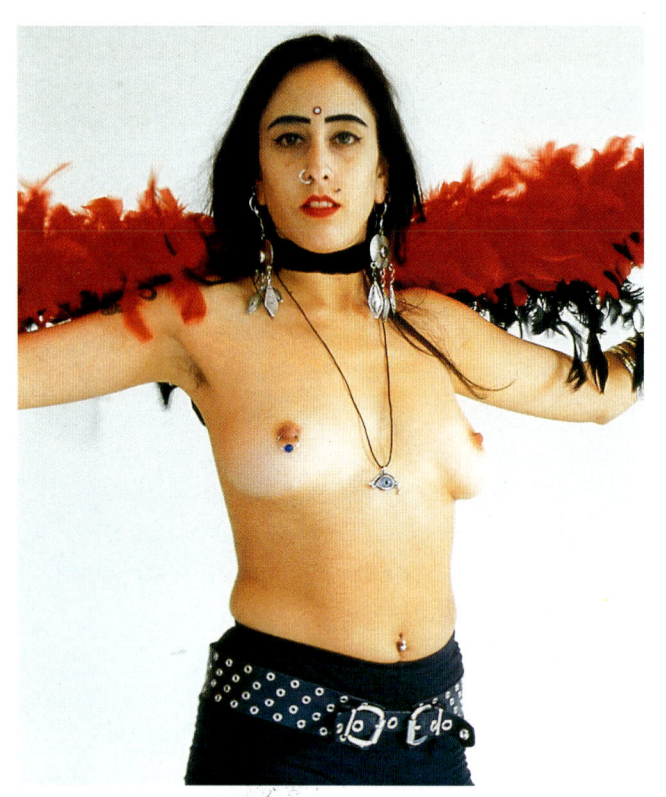

PIERCING MAY NOT ONLY LOOK UNUSUAL, IT CAN ALSO ADD AN EXCITING DIMENSION TO YOUR SEX-LIFE

Many people find earrings attractive, and if you pierce a nipple or penis, you can hang stylish ornaments from them. But looks are not the main reason for the more "serious" forms of body piercing. Those that have such piercings say that they contribute directly to sexual pleasure, by causing the surrounding tissue to become more sensitive and so give greater sensation during sexual arousal. Users also say that tweaking body jewellery produces sexual excitement, even orgasm.

The obvious fear of most people would be that jewellery worn in an intimate spot might get caught or torn out and cause injury to the wearer or their partner. Users say that this does not happen and report that jewellery, if felt at all, adds to their partner's sexual sensations. They add that rings with a proper closure are smooth enough not to damage condoms or diaphragms. However, since using body jewellery has never been part of a scientific study, it would be up to you to decide how you feel about the risks.

It may make you wince to think of a bar or ring being inserted through a tender part of your body, but people who have had it done say it actually feels pleasant. When choosing the site to be pierced, you need to pay attention to the style of your clothing and what you do in your spare time. For example, certain piercings might make bicycle or horse riding uncomfortable, and navel piercings could be troublesome if you tend to wear tight waistbands, as would labia or clitoral piercing if you favour tight jeans.

Leave it to the experts

Having your nipples or genitals pierced is as safe or unsafe as having your ears done. That is, you would be extremely unwise to try to do it yourself and should only be pierced by an experienced professional. They should be registered with the local Health Authority to do such work and should only do the piercing with properly sterilized instruments. This means that the instruments should be correctly treated in an autoclave, not just given a quick dunk in a disinfectant, or come ready-packed in sealed units marked as being sterile. You can now have your ears done with a disposable gun that comes ready-packed, sterilized and loaded with a stud or ring. These are not suitable for nipple or genital piercing, so a special hollow piercing needle must be employed. If proper hygiene is followed, you will not be at risk of infection, but do choose your piercer carefully.

PILLOW BOOKS IN BANGKOK, READERS' WIVES IN BERLIN

Books have been a form of sex aid since our ancestors first started making something a bit more portable than a painting on a cave wall. The Chinese had "Pillow Books" – text and pictures of lovemaking that lovers could read together and imitate. Far from being considered pornographic, such books were seen as an essential part of the arts of love.

In the West, people tend to believe that sex is supposed to be a private event, but the fact is that most of us can be interested or aroused by the thought, sight or sound of other people's bodies and other people's sexual activities. We may like something that can fuel our private fantasies; we may need a reminder to get ourselves or a partner going; we may want specific ideas or suggestions. Whatever, using sexy pictures of other people, or ourselves, is pretty common around the world, in spite of different cultural responses to the respectability of such behaviour. Belgium is the only country never to have censored sexy films.

A comparatively new western European trend, however, is that of "Readers' Wives". Couples have probably been making photographs and films

Mirror, mirror on the wall...

Try watching yourselves making love by placing a mirror in a strategic spot. Mirrors on the bedroom wall can be set to show the two of you on the bed from various angles. If you don't want visitors to guess what you are up to, put the mirror on the inside of a wardrobe door and leave the door ajar when you go to bed. Or get a mirror on a stand, and just wheel it out of the way when not in use. If you would like to cover a wider area, try putting mirror tiles or reflective paper across a whole wall, or on the ceiling.

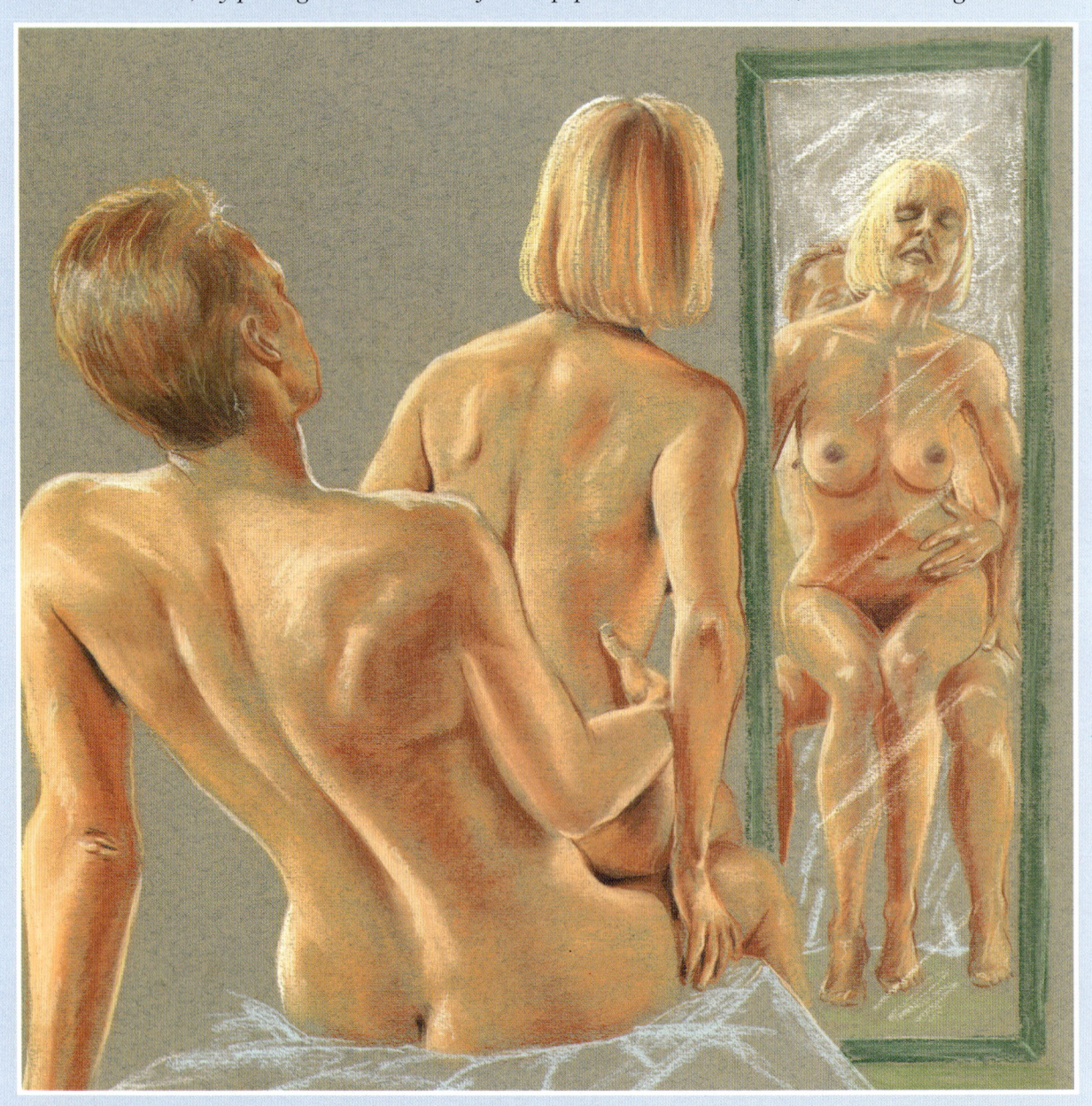

DOUBLE YOUR FUN BY USING A MIRROR TO SEE YOURSELVES IN ACTION

of each other in sexually explicit poses for as long as we have had the technology. What may be new is the number of couples now offering these for general view, in magazines or as videos available on the general market. Being watched can be as exciting as being the spectator. In parts of the world where privacy is an important aspect of lovemaking, there is an extra thrill for many people in breaking that taboo.

There is a common myth in the West that women are not as aroused by pornography as men. Recent studies are beginning to show that women can be just as turned on by exciting matter as men can. Providing, that is, the sexual material is attractive to women.

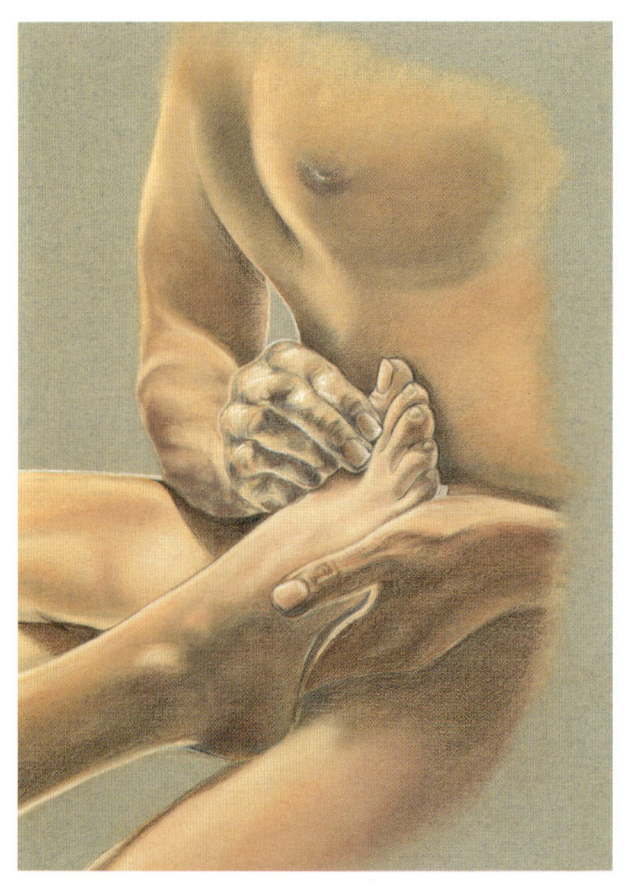

PORNOGRAPHY SHOULD NEVER BE EXPLOITATIVE. MANY PEOPLE ARE EXCITED BY SEEING OTHER PEOPLE HAVING SEX, BUT THE SENSUAL STROKING OF A FOOT CAN BE JUST AS EROTIC TO WATCH AS "HARD-CORE" SEXUAL ACTS

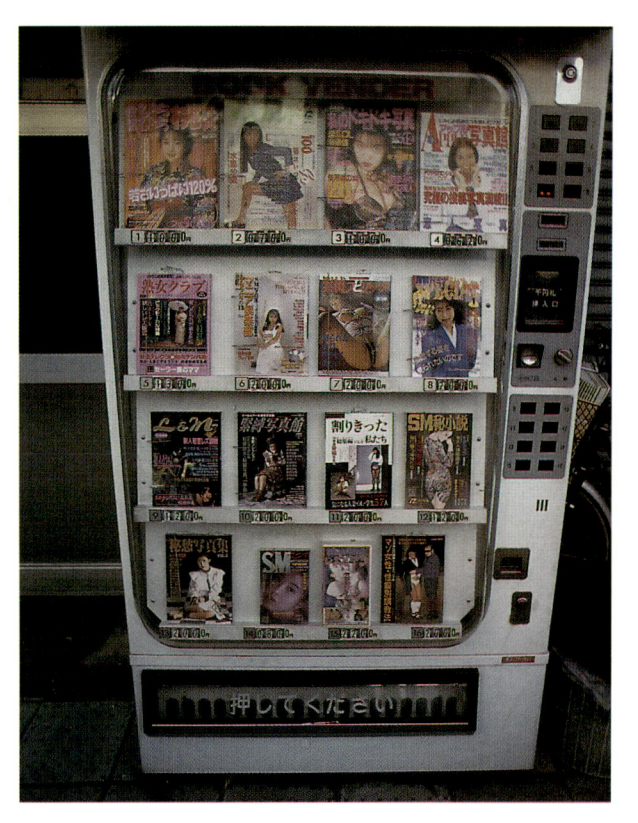

IN SOME COUNTRIES, YOU DON'T EVEN HAVE TO GO TO THE NEWSAGENT FOR YOUR SEXY PUBLICATIONS – THEY ARE WIDELY AVAILABLE FROM VENDING MACHINES AT THE DROP OF A COIN

Women are often revolted by pornography, not because erotic material in itself is unappetizing, but because the material offered is unappealing. What is "wrong" with the vast majority of current pornography is that it shows sex from an entirely male point of view. Women are presented, not as people with whom one shares lovemaking, but as objects with which a man can achieve excitement and orgasm. The important element that makes an item erotic rather than pornographic, that makes a sexual act a true and equal exchange rather than abusive, is that neither person is there simply for the use of the other.

There is a belief that pornography corrupts and degrades and that viewing it will lead to sexual abuse. These fears are often fuelled by rape and child sexual abuse cases where the men and women involved claim that it was reading or seeing pornography that drove them to commit the abuse in the first place. The evidence is very far from clear, however. It could just as reasonably be claimed that a society that allows the circulation of pornography showing women as objects, to be used by men purely for their sexual satisfaction, is actively encouraging sex crimes. But it could also be argued that any rapist who puts the blame on pornography could simply be attempting to shift responsibility for their own actions.

When the Danes decriminalized pornography in 1969, sex crimes fell, dramatically in some categories. It should also be remembered that sexually explicit material is seen every day by millions of people who do not rape or abuse. All kinds of cultures make such material a part of their love-lives, and always have. The Japanese, for instance, have an astoundingly low incidence of rape, yet violently explicit popular comics are available at every bookstall.

So, we've looked at love and courtship around the world, at sexual positions and techniques and sexual aids of various sorts. Every culture has its areas of sexual taboo, areas in which sexual behaviour may be seen as unacceptable or illegal, and these are very different from one society to the next. Paying for sex and gender choices are just two of the areas that we will be exploring in the next chapter, as we consider that one person's poison may be another's meat!

There are many countries where sex can easily be found for sale in tolerated "red light" districts, and sometimes, with a few restrictions only, in legally allowed brothels. Customers may tour these areas openly, window-shopping and viewing the wares on sale before making their purchase

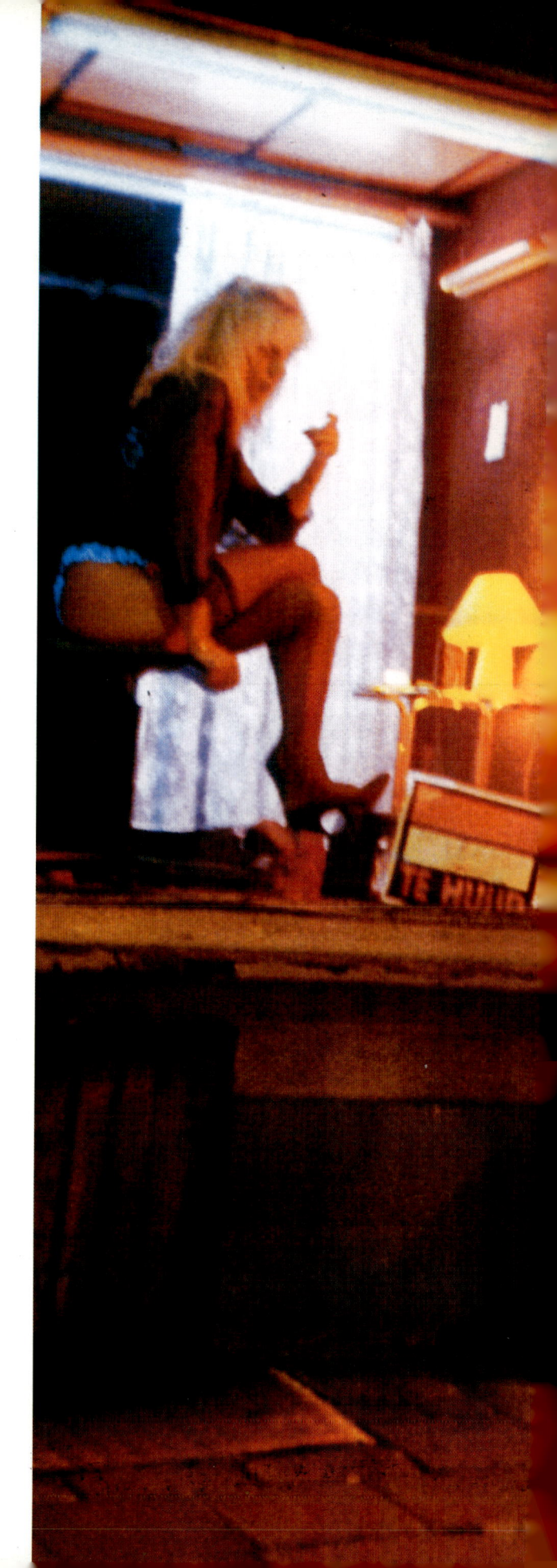

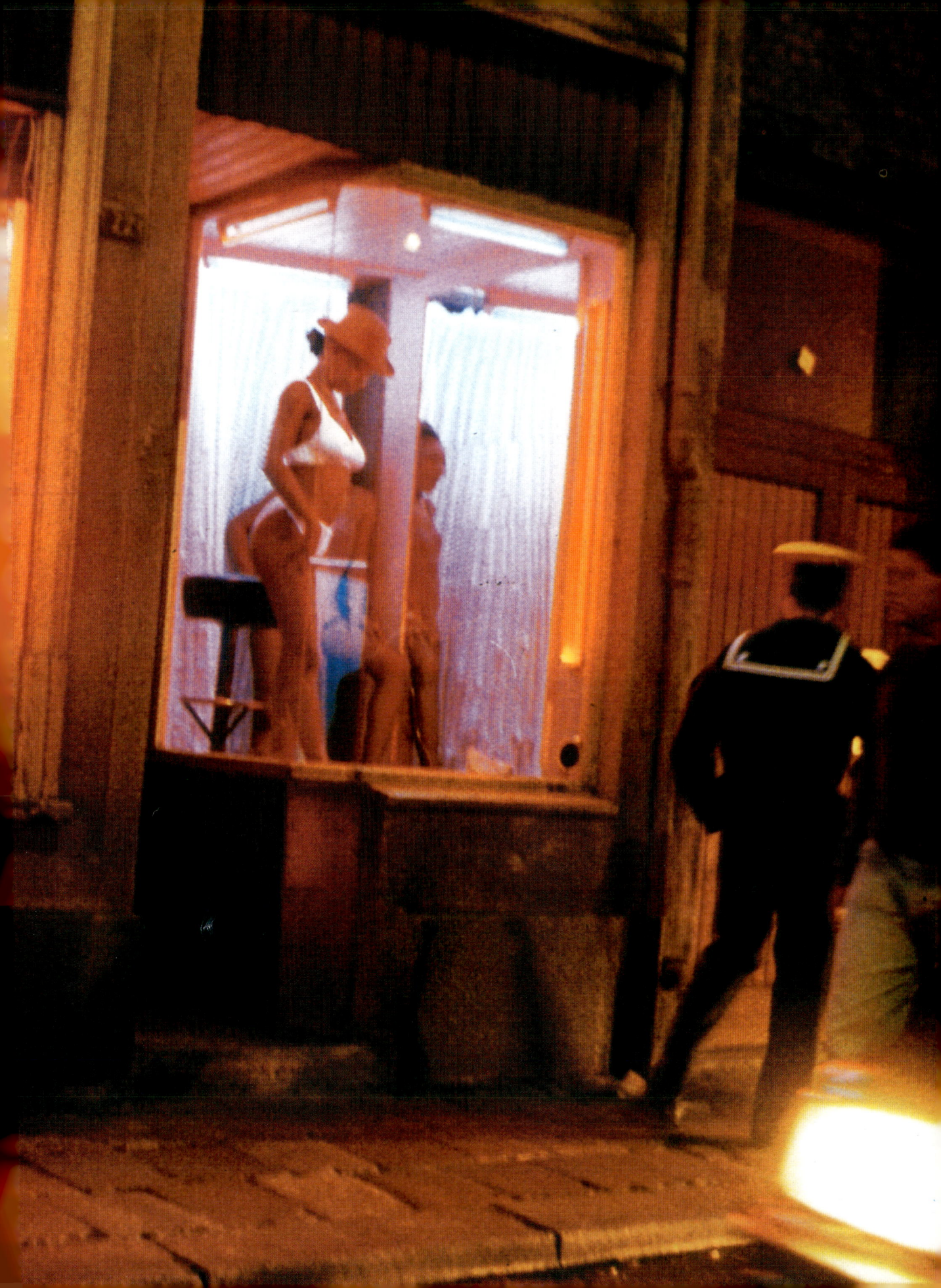

Vive les *differences*

Every human society has different expectations about what sort of sexual practices are normal and what are abnormal. Something taboo in one culture may be positively encouraged or be essential in another. For instance, in some societies a man can be put to death for having sex with another man and the Fang of Africa believe that homosexual behaviour will be punished with leprosy. In other cultures, however, sex between men is either tolerated or considered totally acceptable and an essential part of growing up normally. All males of the Siwans of Africa have sex with other men and among the Tiswana in Botswana, co-wives frequently have sex together when their husbands are away and there is no taboo against it.

Different cultures have a different spin on sex, but adornment and display are found everywhere

VIVE LES DIFFERENCES

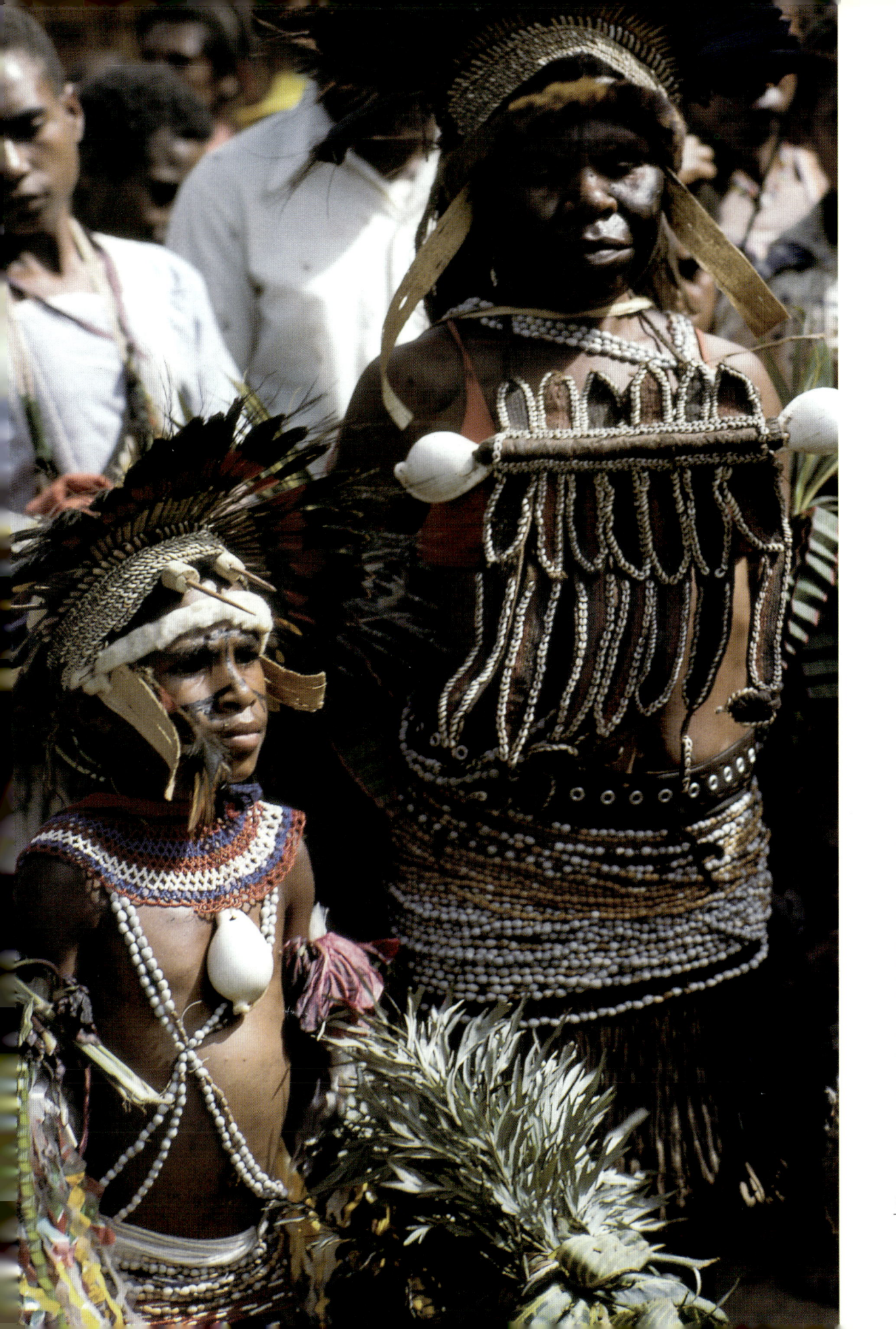

Taking it like a man

The Etoro of Oceania require boys to engage in sex-play with their elders during their initiation education. They think that, because boys have no semen at birth, they have to acquire it before puberty, or be infertile as men. Their belief is that a boy gathers all the semen he will need as a man by having oral sex with mature men. In New Guinea, the Karaki also expect their boys to have anal intercourse with older men during puberty rites and indeed believe they will not grow up normally unless they have received the semen of others. Since they also think that men can get pregnant, part of the ceremony involves eating limes, which are supposed to have contraceptive properties.

HOMOSEXUALITY

Homosexuality appears in all societies around the globe. What is interesting is that it would seem that the percentage of gay men and women present in all cultures is similar, regardless of whether that society is totally tolerant or totally intolerant of homosexuality. What's more, all societies seem to produce the same continuum of homosexual behaviour. That is, ranging from men and women who occasionally have sex with their own gender, through bi-sexuality where a person has same-sex as often as opposite-sex contacts, to men and women who only have sex with their own gender. Even more extraordinary, gay men and women in all societies do, to an extent, resemble each other in mannerisms and behaviour.

In the West, we tend to think of homosexuality as a clearly defined state; you either are or you are not gay. In many other societies, however, it's just considered to be an unremarkable part of normal behaviour. Men and women have sexual relationships with members of their own sex at times and this is not felt to be abnormal. Nor is it necessarily part of a relationship at all. In New Guinea, men have sex with younger male partners without love or romance being part of it.

LESBIANISM

Far less is known about female than male homosexuality around the world. An early study on cultural attitudes towards homosexuality found that 64% of societies examined considered at least some male homosexual acts to be normal and acceptable for certain members of the community, but only five societies specifically approved of lesbianism. This may be partly because homosexuality has a certain part to play in societies where men are in charge and women are often secluded from them until after marriage. In such situations, men may turn to each other for sex-play, but usually in a way that mimics later male/female relationships – for example, an older man who takes the lead role with a young boy.

In many groups (those dominated by men, some would say), what happens between women is simply not considered to be part of the mainstream of social behaviour, so, however much it may happen, it simply isn't talked about. It does tend to be reported more often in societies where men have multiple wives, especially where these wives live together, apart from men. In societies in which the sexes have more equality, such as parts of Europe and the USA, it would appear that as many women as men feel themselves to be gay or bi-sexual.

Most Mexican men have sex with both men and women. Instead of dividing people into three categories – homo, hetero and bi-sexual – they see people as falling into one of nine roles. These depend on what sort of sex they have and whether they have sex mainly with other men or with women or with both. Sexual orientation isn't seen as being based on whether a man has sex with

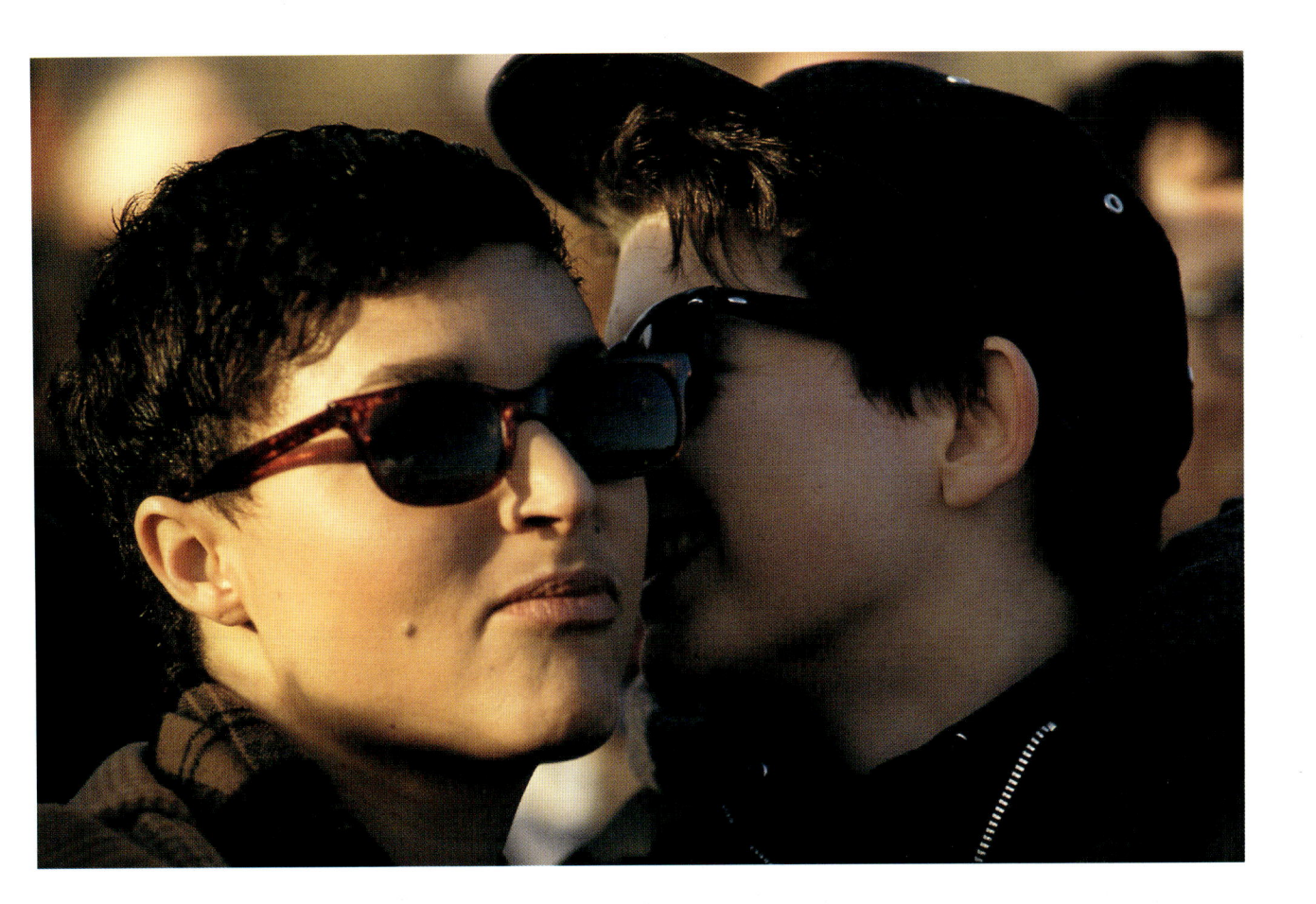

ONE OF THE BIGGEST RECENT CHANGES IN THE WEST HAS BEEN THE RISING TOLERANCE OF GAY SEX, AND COUPLES NOW FEEL MORE ABLE TO SHOW AFFECTION FOR THEIR LOVERS OPENLY

another man but whether he is active or passive when he does. What's more, anal sex is fairly common in Mexico, both as a form of birth control and as a way of retaining virginity. Because anal sex is common between men and women, having anal sex with a man is not as despised as in a society such as Britain, where it is quite a taboo.

In Brazil, Turkey, Algeria and in many other parts of the Middle East, men are only considered to be homosexual if they play the passive role. A passive male partner in gay sex is considered to have less status than a non-passive man or a woman, but homosexual men are not faced with the sort of homophobic fear and anger they still find in Europe and North America.

In some societies, cross-gender sexual behaviour is seen to be evidence of an entirely different sort of individual who is a unique sexual and social being – a third sex. The Navaho, for instance, consider there to be three sexes – male, female and *nadleeh*. "Men" and "women" can be nadleeh. A family in which a nadleeh is born is considered very lucky, since Navaho mythology says that, when humankind was created, the nadleeh were entrusted with all the wealth. A family with a nadleeh is assured financial success.

Native American nations, particularly in the north-west, have a tradition of the *berdache*. This is a male transvestite who acts as a woman in every way. A berdache dresses as a woman, performs female tasks and has sexual relationships with men, often indeed becoming a wife. In some societies, in Korea, Vietnam, Indonesia, Borneo,

New Mexico and Siberia, transvestite men often serve as shamans or priests – the wise person who cares for the group and has been chosen to stand between them and the gods.

In some societies, it is common for men to marry boys who have been brought up in a female role. In Greenland, some boys are brought up as transvestites called *achnutshik*, and they become the wives of another man when puberty arrives. Among the Nambutji in Australia, when a young man reaches the age of twelve, he becomes the boy-wife of an older man. When he gets to eighteen, his "husband" performs his circumcision at his coming of age celebration. As he gets older, he marries his "husband's" daughter. Throughout the six years that he spends learning to be a man, he has an active sexual relationship with his husband and mentor.

MALE MARRIAGE

In Siberia, a berdache is called a *chukchee*. A berdache can be legally married to a man and may also have a wife of their own. Among the Koniag people of North America, certain boys are raised to be female and are then married to important members of the community because they are considered to have special, magical powers.

Northern Europe, particularly in its English- and German-speaking cultures, is unique in the pattern of its homosexuality. In other cultures, man-on-man relationships either involve an adult man and a young boy, such as in New Guinea, or a man with an adult man who takes on the clothing and mannerisms of a woman, such as the berdache of North America or the *hijra* of India. Only in northern Europe and in areas where Europeans have migrated, such as the United States, does it involve two adults neither of whom tries to change their sex role.

Touching bases

If one man touches another man's penis, it doesn't necessarily mean he's making a pass. From very early times it's been a common custom in many cultures to swear an oath by putting your hand on a man's most treasured possession. The Walbiri of central Australia have a novel form of saying hello, because instead of shaking hands, they shake penes.

DRESSING UP

Cross-dressing, or transvestism, is perhaps the most obvious form of sexual behaviour where one culture's taboo is another culture's institution. In the West, the accepted definition of a TV or transvestite is a man with a compulsion to dress like or otherwise personify a woman while still accepting a male identity. In essence, it is seen as a sexual disorder. A typical transvestite would be a man who appears quite normal at all times when he is not cross-dressing. He is not likely to be homosexual, will prefer women as his sex partners and will most certainly not want to lose his penis. In contrast, a typical male transexual will not identify in any way with his male body. He believes that he is a woman and is trapped in the body of a man. To him, his penis is a mistake of Nature and he will want to get rid of it.

Some professionals suggest that there is not a clear distinction between transvestism and transexuality and see it simply as a continuum, with the cross-dressing man being at the

THE *HIJRAS* OF INDIA ARE A DISTINCT GROUP WHO LIVE IN THEIR OWN COMMUNITIES. THEY ARE TRANSVESTITE, TRANSEXUAL, GAY OR BI-SEXUAL; SOME ARE EVEN HERMAPHRODITE. *HIJRAS* ARE WIDELY TOLERATED IN INDIA AND MAY EVEN BE PAID TO ATTEND SOCIAL OCCASIONS SUCH AS WEDDINGS AS THEY ARE THOUGHT TO BRING GOOD LUCK

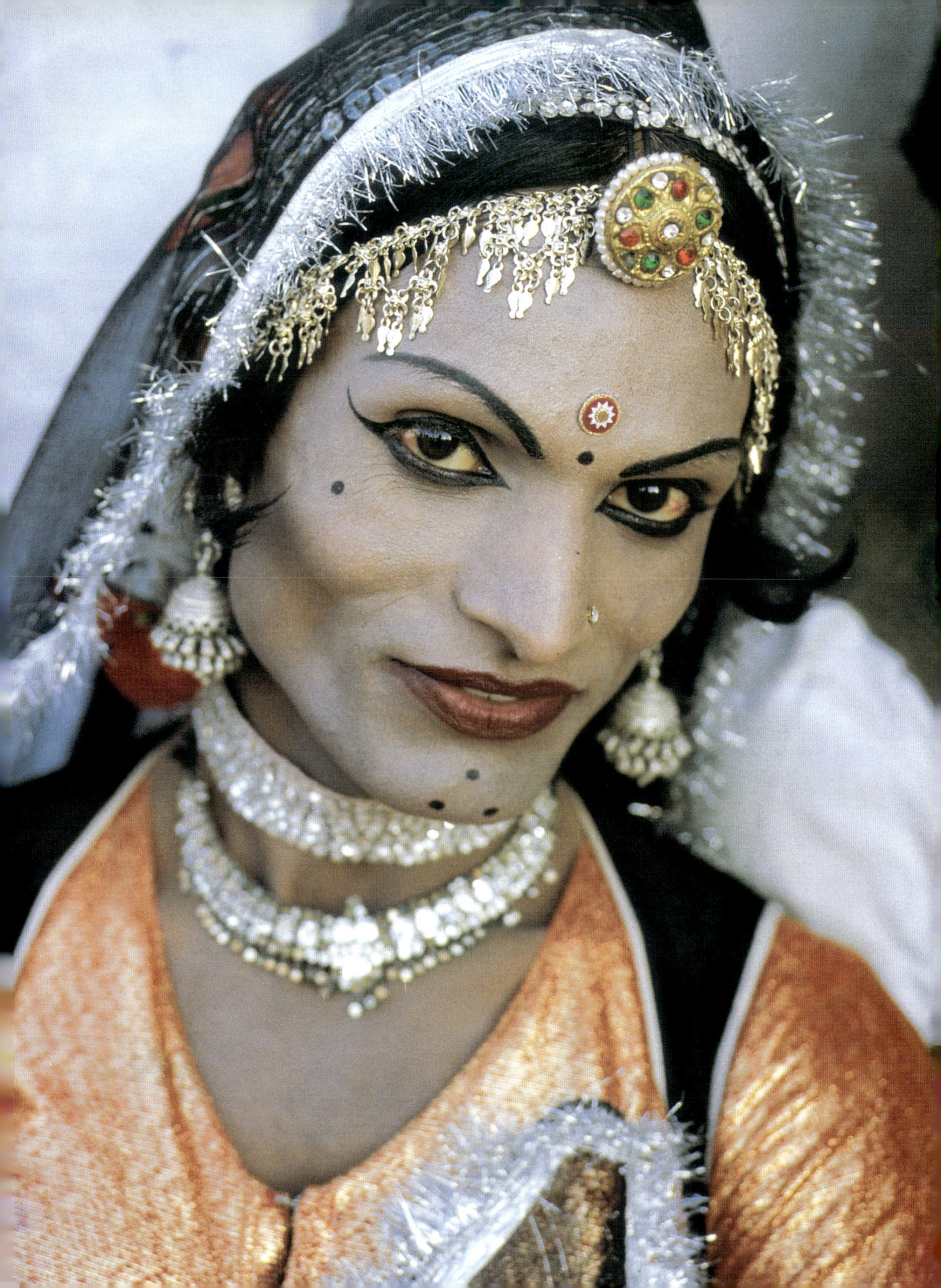

beginning of an ever-increasing identification with the opposite sex.

A lot of the confusion and myth that surrounds transvestism probably comes from the fact that, in the West, it has always had a bad press and attracted hostile public attitudes. Until recently, cross-dressing has been forced into being a very secretive activity. Why do men become cross-dressers? There are a few curious factors to be considered when we look at cross-dressing. For a start, it is a mainly male activity. North American nations have the additional tradition of "manly hearted women", which are women who dress as men and take on roles more usually reserved for men in their cultures. But in other cultures with a transvestite tradition, it is only men who cross the barriers.

Many reasons have been put forward for cross-dressing. For some men, it is a way of challenging society's preconceptions about gender. Some men cross-dress because they are unhappy about being men. Others don't mind the male state, but simply like putting on women's clothes occasionally. Some men cross-dress simply to make a passing social or fashion statement, and some because they have emotional needs that can only be met by the comfort that wearing women's clothes gives them.

But for many transvestites in Europe and North America, cross-dressing is an intensely sexual activity. Most transvestites have their first cross-dressing experience around puberty or in adolescence. The first experience is likely to be sexually exciting and the young person will carry on with the practice. However, transvestism is not just a sexual variation. There have always been plenty of men who get a sexual thrill from their cross-dressing, but the accepted view of most experts in this field is that these are not the majority. Some transvestites do masturbate as part of their cross-dressing routine, and it is easy to see why this is such an attractive prospect. After all, it is like making love to the idealized feminine image you have created for yourself without any fear of the disappointment, criticism or rejection that might come with attempts at intercourse with someone else. However, in most cases, the primary satisfaction is more cerebral – a feeling of comfort, a freeing of tension and intense enjoyment of total control.

Transvestism tends to happen in societies that separate elements of human experience into female or male, insisting that women do one thing and men another, that women feel one way and men another. In plenty of societies, the strict divisions between the sexes can be varied. For instance, men of the North American Zuni never fight over women but their women will certainly come to blows over men. Among the Ojibwa, a woman may be accepted as a hunter or a shaman and if she shows skills in these areas she will be treated as an equal to the men. And in New Guinea, Manu fathers take on total responsibility for bringing up children.

In other cultures, transexual behaviour is accepted for another reason. In societies with a firm idea of what behaviour is appropriate to each sex, the exaggerated "female" behaviour of a transvestite or transexual male can be reassuring and exciting. Men in the Middle East, South America and Italy will often say that TV or TS men are far better at sexually pleasing a man than a "real" woman, and that their style of dress and seduction is more of a turn-on. For this reason, transexual and transvestite prostitutes are as numerous, if not more so, and often more popular, than female prostitutes in these countries. In other societies, homosexual, transvestite or transexual men are not only considered to best understand how to please men but also to be most skilled at passing on those secrets. In Kenya, it is said that some families will engage the services of such a man in order to teach a bride-to-be ways in which she can satisfy her husband.

Sex and gender

SEX is the purely biological element of our sexual identity. That is, it is the chromosomes, hormones and genitalia that make you either a male or a female in physical terms, and will allow you to mature into taking on the male or female role in the sexual act in later years.

GENDER is your sexual identity, which is usually in line with your biological sex. Gender, however, also relates to the various feelings, thoughts, behaviour and fantasies that you have about sexual behaviour. Each society has an idea of what is appropriate for males and females and you are brought up with all kinds of cues, clues, rewards and punishments telling you what being "male" or "female" is all about.

GENDER IDENTITY is our sense of which sex we belong to. For the majority of people, this is a fairly straightforward matter. Most children will have the confirmed conviction that they are undoubtedly a boy or a girl by about the age of three and this conviction about their "core" gender identity will tend to stay more or less constant for the rest of their lives.

GENDER ROLE is the public face of your personal gender identity. That is, everything that you say or do that indicates to those around you to what degree you are either "male" or "female". From the feedback you get, you might be made to adjust your own gender identity. There is obviously an acceptable gender role in every society and we all learn and internalize these from our earliest years.

CHOOSING THE SEX OF YOUR CHILD

Given the fact that we consider little boys and little girls to be different, not just in the shape of their bits but in the status this gives them, it's hardly surprising that many people around the world have a preference for the sex of their children. Several cultures believe that it all has to do with right or left testicles. Sperm from the right testicle give boys, those from the left give girls. In the 19th century, the French nobility would have the left testicle surgically removed to guarantee a son. Pacific islanders thought that a woman need do no more than swap clothes with her mate when they settled down to make love, to make a boy baby.

We live in a world in which most cultures apportion behaviour, traits and power according to your sex. Which means that most would-be parents express a choice for the sex of a child. It may be for a girl, "to look after us in our old age", or a boy, "to help in the family business". Whichever, the ideal family in some cultures is often described as being two children, one of each sex. But in many others, girls are seen as a financial burden while boys are not only valuable as workers and wage-earners, they are status-bringers and essential to some aspects of religious observance.

When she is left to her own devices, Nature has a remarkably balanced view on how many of each sex there should be. All things being equal, there is a man for every woman, an Adam for every Eve. About 105 boys are born to every 100 girls, but there is a slightly higher rate of infant death and miscarriage amongst boy babies. And whether or not you believe in the Gaia theory that our planet is a self-regulating organism, there does seem to be a mechanism in Nature that takes account of anything that upsets this even balance of the sexes. Two examples of this are that more boys are born during and after major wars, and that population-reducing disasters such as major earthquakes, flood, fire or famine are often followed by a distinct rise in female births.

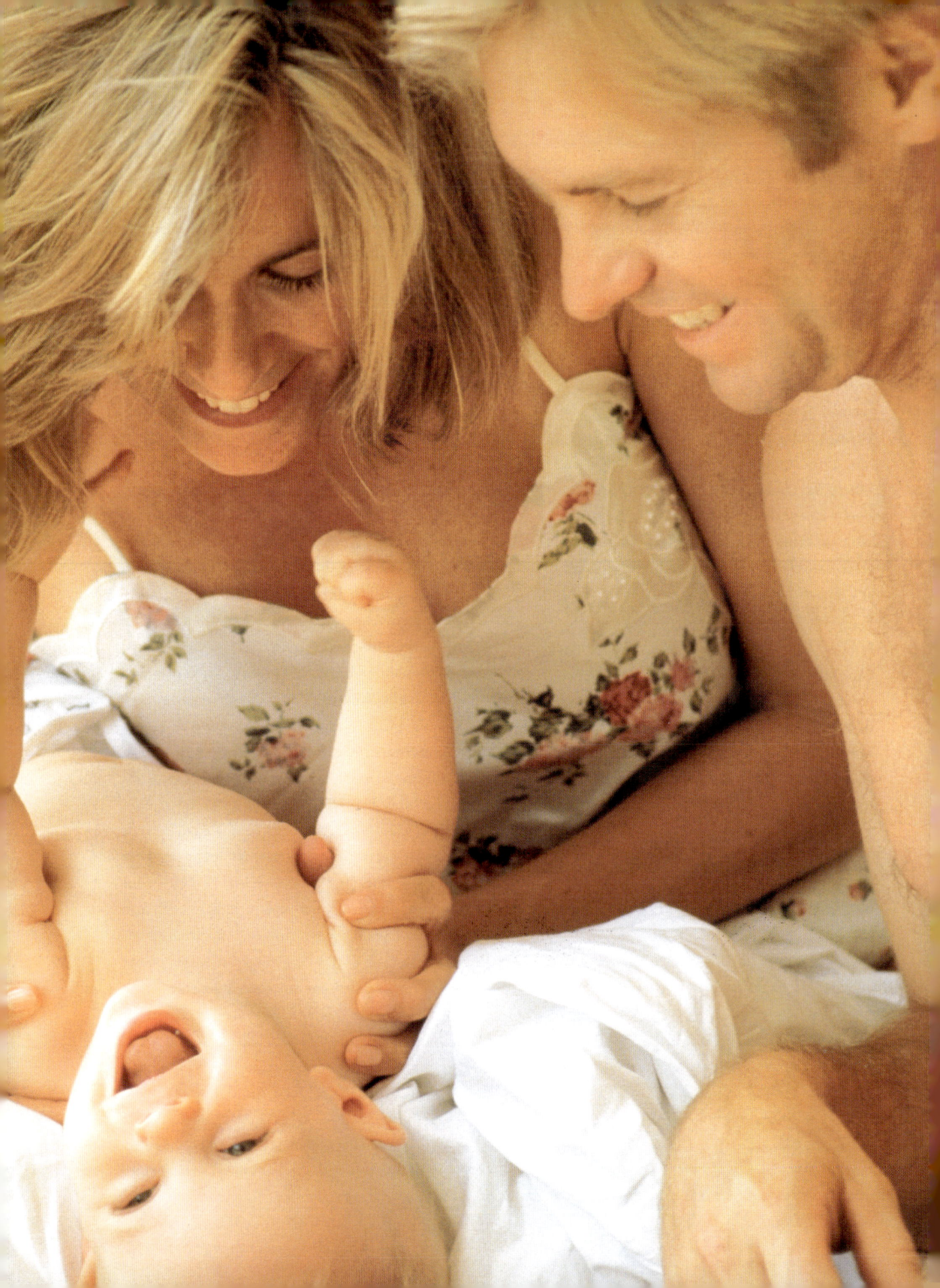

Spin-offs from research into in vitro fertilization have given scientists the potential ability to offer certainty of sex determination. But would it be ethical and sensible to make this technology available for this purpose?

To understand exactly what science is now able to influence, we need to have a close look at what is inside the two essentials in sex determination – the sperm and the egg. All body cells have a nucleus, the cell's control centre and information-giver. The nucleus contains chromosomes, which are strands of the nucleic acid known as DNA. All ordinary body cells contain 46 of these chromosomes, arranged in 23 pairs, 22 of which are identical. The twenty-third pair is the sex chromosomes, which determine gender. In females, this pair can only be matching (termed XX). In males, the pair is made of two different chromosomes (termed X and Y).

Sperm and egg have a nucleus like any other body cell, in the head of a sperm and in the centre of an egg. The crucial difference from other body cells is that a process called "meiosis" ensures that sperm and egg only contain half sets of chromosomes, with 23 singles instead of 23 pairs. When meiosis takes place in a male, the complete double set of chromosomes splits up to make a single set with an X chromosome and a single set with a Y chromosome. Sperm is therefore either X- or Y-carrying. Since, as explained above, women can only have matching XX chromosomes, meiosis in turn can only produce half sets with an X, so all eggs are X-carrying. When a sperm penetrates an egg, their two half sets of chromosomes come together at fertilization to form a set of 46 chromosomes. If a Y type sperm does the deed, then the XY result will be a potential boy, and if it is an X type, the XX result will be a potential girl.

NEW TECHNOLOGY MAY MAKE IT POSSIBLE FOR YOU TO CHOOSE THE SEX OF YOUR CHILD – IS THIS A GOOD THING?

Science's ability to influence the sex of a baby is the result of work that was initially considered to be for preventing hereditary conditions from being passed on, for improving animal breeding or for immunology. If we put aside the ethical and social implications and simply consider how we could guarantee the sex of a child, it would be by perfecting techniques in these three areas:

- *Immunizing the woman against either X or Y sperm.*
- *Using Artificial Insemination after first separating the X and Y sperm.*
- *Changing the conditions in the woman's vagina and cervix so that only Y sperm or only X sperm would pass on to a rendezvous with an egg.*

Immunization is when the body's defences are marshalled against an intruder. It might be possible to make an X- or Y-bearing sperm appear as such, although nothing has been found so far that could make the body distinguish in this way between the two different types of sperm.

It seems logical that if you could separate male-producing from female-producing sperm and use the sperm of choice for artificial fertilization, you would have a 100% effective route for choosing the sex of a baby. At present, researchers in the United States have claimed an 80% success rate in producing male rather than female babies using the separation method. Their method is supposed to sort Y-bearing from X-bearing sperm by filtering sperm through protein. However, other scientists are sceptical about these results.

One method that can be used to positively identify X from Y sperm is to use the dye quinacrine, which reacts with a spot found only on Y chromosomes and can be shown up under ultraviolet light. Alas, this is not the answer since it also kills sperm. However, using some sort of dye does seem to be the main hope for the future in this field.

The problem is hard to solve because the only difference agreed so far is that X chromosomes are twice as large as Y. However, this does not mean that X-carrying sperm are twice as large as the Y kind. Research suggests that the separation could possibly be done by using the characteristics of Y sperm being fast-swimming but short-lived, while X are slow-swimming and longer-living. However, statistics from clinics in the States suggest that such separation methods are not particularly reliable. There is also the fear that any couple desperate enough to go to these sort of lengths may be tempted to abort if the method failed and the foetus was identified as the "wrong sex".

Currently, there are three ways that the sex of a foetus can be detected. The commonest method is amniocentesis, which involves drawing off a little of the amniotic fluid in which the developing baby is floating. This can only be done after 16 weeks of the pregnancy. A newer test, chorionic biopsy, involves drawing off cells from the inside of the womb. This can be done between the sixth and tenth weeks of a pregnancy. Both of these tests involve examining chromosomes and are primarily intended as ways of checking for abnormalities such as Down's Syndrome. They are not entirely risk-free, and medical ethics would probably stop most doctors from offering tests purely for the purpose of sexing a baby, but this information might be given on request if you had the tests for other reasons. The third testing technique, scanning, is risk-free. Some experts claim they can use this to tell the sex of a baby from as early as 16 weeks, but most operators would admit that it has to be much further on in a pregnancy for certainty.

In countries where sex selection is culturally very important, an imbalance in the sexes is beginning to emerge. China adopted a "one child, one family" policy some years ago, in response to the country's overpopulation problem. The result, unfortunately, seems to have been an unusual number of sons being born. There is speculation that girl babies are aborted, or die soon after birth, so that couples wanting a son can try again without incurring the penalties of having more than one child. In India too, girls have a higher chance of being aborted or not surviving to adulthood.

What you can do

If you want to try for a boy or a girl, you could at least consider these ideas. Y sperm are faster-swimming but have less stamina and X are the reverse. Vaginal fluid affects sperm – the more alkaline it is, the more it favours male-carrying sperm and the more acidic, the better it is for female.
So, if you want a girl you could:
- *Make the vagina mildly acidic with a teaspoon of white vinegar to a pint of water douche just before having sex.*
- *Try to avoid the woman having an orgasm, as this makes the vagina and cervix more alkaline.*
- *Disadvantage the shorter-lived Y sperm by having your intended baby-making intercourse a day or so before ovulation.*
- *Make the stronger-swimming Y sperms' job harder and their journey longer by ejaculating just inside the vagina.*

If you want a boy:
- *Douche with bicarbonate of soda.*
- *Have sex at or immediately after ovulation.*
- *Have deep penetration.*
- *Have an orgasm!*

Finally, as a last resort, you could try to fit in with some of the statistics:
- *More boys are born during the first year and a half of marriage.*
- *First babies are more often boys.*
- *Mid-year is the peak period for male births.*
- *You are more likely to have girls the more children you have.*
- *More daughters are born to older parents.*
- *Fertility treatment drugs are more likely to result in girls.*

Paying for it

Who pays for sex? Christian and Islamic societies tend to disapprove of prostitution. People in Britain, for example, consider it the last resort of the sexually incompetent. Prostitution has a very different reputation in other parts of the world.

A study in Colombia showed that 65% of men in college had visited a prostitute and in a study in Naples, a third of men had had at least one sexual encounter with a prostitute in the previous six months. In Japan, hostesses, bar girls and call girls in the tradition of the elegant geisha are all still a part of the social structure. A night on the town for a group of well-to-do businessmen is quite likely to include paying for sex.

In many cultures, prostitutes are excluded from "polite society". Not so among the Hausa people of West Africa. There, a head prostitute is crowned with a turban and installed in her office in a public ceremony.

JAPAN HAS A LONG TRADITION OF PAYING FOR FEMALE COMPANY. GEISHAS HAVE A REPUTATION IN THE WEST FOR THEIR SEXUAL SKILLS, BUT MAY OFTEN SIMPLY PROVIDE COMPANIONSHIP

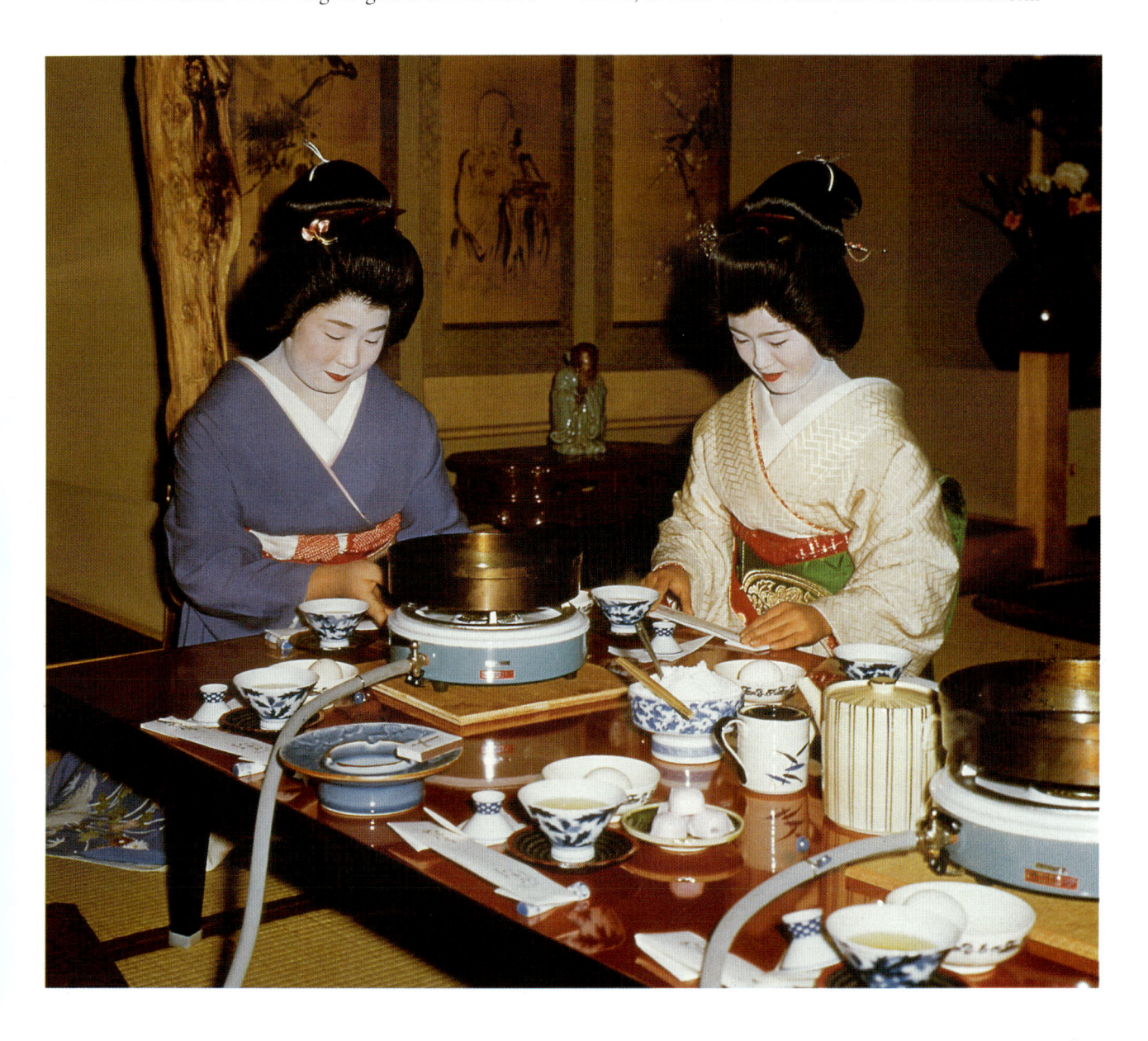

Prostitution

In some cultures, there is simply no notion of the concept of prostitution. However, women may quite normally and naturally expect the men with whom they have sex to give them presents, and the men expect to have to do so. This is so among the Trobriand Islanders but no one considers that this is a form of prostitution.

SURFIN' THE NET FOR SATISFACTION

Once upon a time, there were highly suggestive cave paintings, then there were pillow books, then there were raunchy magazines and videos. The hi-tech version is what you will find available now on floppy discs, CD-ROMs or through the Internet, which basically offer games and "literature". If you have a personal computer, your sexual habits can be brought into the 21st century with high-tech versions of:

1) *"Reading" about sex.*
2) *Making contact with other people.*

In any newsagents you will find magazines for adults only that can introduce you to what is available on PC of a strictly sexual nature. If you have access to the Internet, you'll find that there is even more. By electronic mail you can receive text, pictures, video and sound from anywhere around the world. What is possible at the moment is to have an interactive encounter in real time or with a programme that will put someone on your screen who will perform the actions you dictate. Interactive computer sex originated in America, but the Japanese probably have the largest range of interactive porn available at the moment. On the Internet, it's as easy to call the other side of the world as the other side of your street and it gives you the opportunity to gossip with, chat up and even date, in reality or in fantasy, other Internet users. There have already been several relationships and marriages between people who have met in this way.

Coming soon – and sooner than you may think – is virtual reality sex. At the moment, visual messages are all you can receive on a computer. But already, work is being done on translating the other senses. A body suit is in development that will allow you to feel the sensations a programme or another person sends to you – the ultimate in safer sex. With the Internet, global sex may soon be only a phone call away, and all the diverse ways of making love will be at your fingertips.

The language of love

If you want to explore more International Good Sex, remember the two necessities. One is a condom! The other is those three little words, in the language of your destination. Just to start you off, here they are, in:

ENGLISH: *I love you*
ESPERANTO: *Mi amas vin*
FRENCH: *Je t'aime*
GERMAN: *Ich liebe dich*
ITALIAN: *Ti amo*
SPANISH: *Te amo*
SWEDISH: *Jag alskar dig*
DUTCH: *Ik hou van je*
JAPANESE: *Aishite masu*
ARABIC: *Ana b hebek*

TODAY, SEX FOR MANY PEOPLE IS A MATTER OF GETTING CLOSER TO THEIR PARTNERS. BUT WITH RAPIDLY DEVELOPING COMMUNICATIONS SYSTEMS SUCH AS THE INTERNET, INCREASING NUMBERS MAY SOON BE GETTING CLOSER TO PEOPLE THOUSANDS OF MILES AWAY – ON THE OTHER SIDE OF THE WORLD!

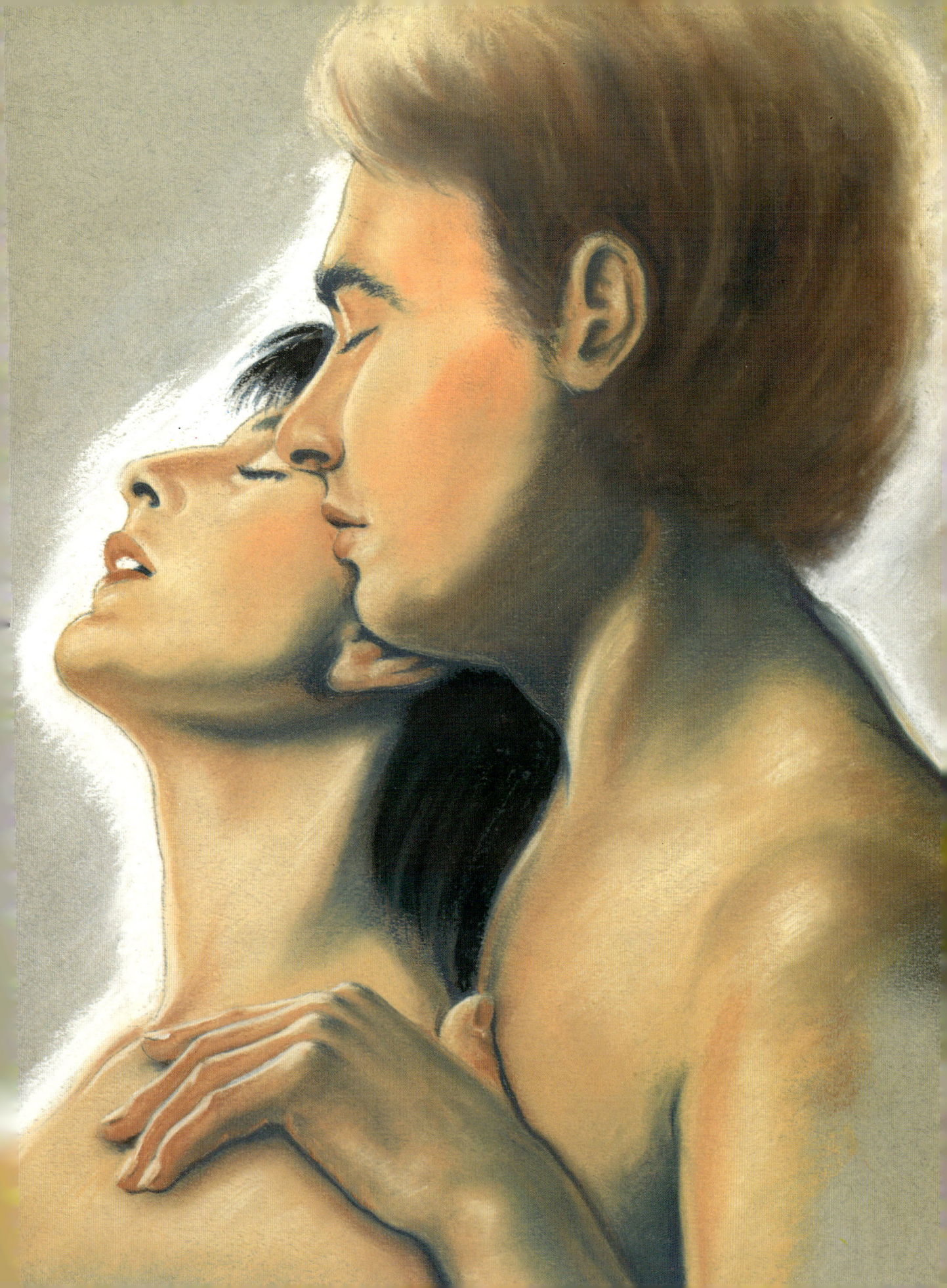

All page numbers in italics refer to illustrations

A

Africa: attractiveness in 13, 18, 21; chastity in 48; children in 39; kissing in 46-7; circumcision in 95, 96; marriage in 32, 35, 36,37; 38, 39 masturbation in 20; nudity in 25; oral sex in 83; premarital sex in 31-2; prostitution in 123; sex toys in 103; sexual characteristics in 15, 40; sexual initiation in 28-29; sexual practices in 56, 59, 86; sexual taboos in 46; sexual techniques in 72, 74; tattoos in 18, 101; virginity in 44, 48
Ananga Ranga 66, 74
aphrodisiacs 98-100
Arabian Nights, The 13
aromatherapy 100-1
Asia: kissing in 47; marriage in 34; sexual positions in 69
attractiveness: in Africa 13, 18, 21; in China 18; in Islam 21; in Japan 21, 24; in men 10, 12, 14; in North America 12, 14; in the Pacific 13; and plastic surgery 94-5; in Western World 9-10, 12, 14-15; in women *9*, 12-23
Australia: sexual practices in 53; sexual techniques in 80

B

bathing 87
books *67*, 68, 75, *76*, 107-8
breasts 15-17, 92, *93*, 94, 97-8
bride abduction 36
bundling 31-2
buttocks 13, 14

C

Chang, Jolan 24
chastity 48
chastity belts 54
children 39, 82
China: aphrodisiacs in 98; attractiveness in 18; marriage in 36; sexual characteristics in 10; sexual practices in 46; sexual taboos in 46; sexual techniques in *45* , 68, 107
circumcision: female 95-6; male 95
clitoris 21-2
clitoral stimulators 104
computers 124
condoms *65*
courtship 31

D

dildos 103

E

ears 24-5
ejaculation 50, 94
Ectomorphs 12
Endomorphs 12
extramarital sex 40, 60-4

F

fetishism 44
food 99
french kissing 47

G

Gautier, Théopile 14
Geishas *123*
gender 119
genital piercing 106-7
genitalia 19-21
gichigich 51
Greece: marriage in 35
group sex 63

H

hair 21, 102
head 23
hijras 116, *117*
homosexuality 114-16
Hormone Replacement Therapy 101
hymen 96-7

I

India: children in 39; hijras in 116, *117* ; marriage in 35, 36, 37; sexual characteristics in 11; sexual taboos in 46
Islam: attractiveness in 21; circumcision in 95, 96; marriage in 34, 35, 40; nudity in 25; prostitution in 123; sexual characteristics in 40; sexual taboos in 46; sexual techniques in 69

J

Japan: attractiveness in 21, 24; Geishas in *123*; prostitution in 123; tattoos in 18
Judaism: circumcision in 95; marriage in 39; sexual practices in 56

K

Kama Sutra, The 11, 49, 66, 75, 76, 80, 91, 106
Kegel, Arnold 94
Kinsey, Alfred 11, 55
kissing 46-7

L

labia 19-20
lesbianism 114
Li T'ung Hsuan 68
love eggs 104

M

marriage *27*, age of 32, *33*, extramarital sex in 40; reasons for 32, 34-5; rituals 38-9; same-sex 40; suitability for 35-6
masturbation 20, 23, 30, 52
men: attractiveness in 10, 12, 14; below partner 77, *78*; circumcision 95; and ejaculation 50; and extramarital sex 40, 63; on top of partner 72-4; sex aids for 90-2, 97
Mesomorphs 12
Mile High Club 86
mirrors *108*
'missionary'-position 72-4
music 53

N

neck 24
night-crawling 31
nipples 17-18, 98
North America: attractiveness in 12, 14; homosexuality in 115-16; sex education in 51; sexual practices in 46; transvestites in 118
nudity 25

O

old age 40-1
oral sex 83, *84-5*
orgasm *21*, 50-1

P

Pacific: attractiveness in 13; circumcision in 95; marriage in 32, 36; masturbation in 20; nudity in 25; oral sex in 83; sex toys in 103; sexual practices in 86; sexual techniques in 51, 72, 80; tattoos in 101; virginity in 44
Papua New Guinea: courtship in 31; genital piercing in 106; sexual aids in 90; sexual practices in 86; sexual techniques in 72
penis 22, 23, 90-2, 97, 106, 116

Perfumed Garden, The 66, 80
pillow books *45*, 107-8
places for sex 86-7
plastic surgery 94-5, 97-8
polyandry 38
polygamy 36-8
pornography 109-10, 124
pregnancy: and sex determination 119-22; and sexual practices 56, *57-8*
premarital sex 31-2
prostitution 123-4

R

'Readers' Wives' 107, 109
rough sex 53-4
Russia: sex education in 51
rear-entry position 68-71

S

sado-masochism 44, 53-4
same-sex marriages 40
sex aids *89*; books 107-8; for men 90-2; mirrors *108*; pornography 109-10
sex determination 119-22
sex education 14, 29-30, 51
sex toys 103-6
sexual characteristics: in Africa 15; in China 10; in India 11; in Islam 40; in Western World 9-10, 40; in women 34
sexual initiation 28-30
sexual positions: 'missionary'-position 72-4; and pregnancy 80-2; rear-entry 68-71; side by side

78; sitting 80; standing 79, 80
sexual practices: in Africa 56, 59, 86; in Australia 53; and childbirth 58-60; in China 45, frequency 55; in Judaism 56; in Papua New Guinea 86; in the Pacific 86; and pregnancy 56, 57-8; places for 86-7; in South America 58; times for 46, 86; in Western World 55, 56, 58-9
sexual taboos 46, 56, 86
sexual techniques: bathing 87; books in 67, 68, 75, 76; mirrors in 108; music in 53; oral sex 83, 84-5; and sex determination 119-22
Sheldon, William 11
shower, use of 80
side by side position 78, 82
sitting position 80, 81
skin 18-19, 101
South America: marriage in 32, 35-6; prostitution in 123; sexual aids in 90; sexual initiation in 28, 30; places for sex 86; sexual practices in 58; sexual taboos in 46; sexual techniques in 71; virginity in 44
Spain: marriage in 34
Spanish Fly 100
standing position 79, 80
swinging 63

T

Tantric sex 47, 50, 51, 94
Tao of Love and Sex, The (Chang) 24
Taoist sex 47, 50
tattoos 18, 101
teeth 18
Thai beads 104
Thailand: sex education in 30
times for sex 46, 86
transexuals 116-18
transvestism 116-18
T'ung Hsuan Tzu (Li) 68

V

vagina 20
vaginal exercises 94
vibrators 103-4
Viravaidya, Mechai 30
virginity 44, 48, 96

W

Western World: attractiveness in 9-10, 12, 14-15; fetishism in 44; hair in 21; homosexuality in 116; marriage in 37-8, 40; masturbation in 30; nudity in 25; premarital sex in 31-2; sado-masochism in 44; sex education in 29-30; sexual characteristics in 10, 40; sexual initiation in 29-30; sexual practices in 44, 55, 56, 58-9; sexual taboos in 46; transvestites in 118
women: attractiveness in 9, 12-23; below partner 74; circumcision 95-6; and extramarital sex 40, 63; and kissing 47; and lesbianism 114; and plastic surgery 97-8; and pornography 109-10; and pregnancy 56; sex toys for 103-4, 105; sexual characteristics 34; on top of partner 77, 78

The publishers would like to thank the following sources for their kind permission to reproduce the pictures in this book: AKG London Ltd/Natural History Museum, Vienna/ Erich Lessing; The Bridgeman Art Library/Victoria Lownes Collection; Robert Butcher; Camera Press/Sally Griffyn, Benoit Gysembergh; Robert Harding Picture Library/David Beatty, Michael Legge, Robert Hanbury-Tenison; The Hutchison Library/Jon Burbank, Michael MacIntyre, Sarah Murray, André Singer; Prospect Pictures; Rex Features; Frank Spooner Pictures/Sion Touhig; Tony Stone Images/Bruce Ayres, Carol Ford; Zefa.

Every effort has been made to acknowledge correctly and contact the source and/or copyright holder of each picture, and Carlton Books Limited apologises for any unintentional errors or omissions which will be corrected in future editions of this book.